AF556718

Library of Congress Cataloging-in-Publication Data

Andrews. Brian T.
Traumatic transtentorial herniation and its management / by Brian T. Andrews, Lawrence H. Pitts.
p. cm.
Includes index.
ISBN 0-87993-383-6 $40.00
1. Traumatic tentorial herniation. I. Pitts, Lawrence H. II. Title.
RD594.A53 1990
617.4'8101—dc20 90-44470
CIP

Copyright © 1991
Futura Publishing Company, Inc.

Published by
Futura Publishing Company, Inc.
2 Bedford Ridge Road
Mount Kisco, New York 10549

L.C. No.: 90-44470
ISBN No.: 0-87993-3836

Every effort has been made to ensure that the information in this book is as up to date and accurate as possible at the time of publication. However, due to the constant developments in medicine, neither the author, nor the editor, nor the publisher can accept any legal or any other responsibility for any errors or omissions that may occur.

All rights reserved.
No part of this book may be translated or reproduced in any form without written permission of the publisher.

Printed in the United States of America

Foreword

Transtentorial herniation is a dreaded sequel of expanding intracranial mass lesions. Although not always possible, it is better to prevent transtentorial herniation than to treat it. This is particularly true in patients with post-traumatic intracranial hematomas because the occurrence of transtentorial herniation and brain stem compression in these patients has an especially deleterious effect on outcome.

In the past 15 years, neurosurgeons have realized the importance of preventing transtentorial herniation and controlling intracranial pressure to maximize the likelihood of a good outcome. Rapid, effective, and rational treatment of impending increase of intracranial pressure and transtentorial herniation is central to the care of the severely head-injured patient.

The title of this book would suggest a narrow focus on transtentorial herniation. However, the authors have endeavored to interpret the title in its broadest sense. This volume reviews the latest advances in the management of severely head-injured patients with specific reference to the diagnosis and treatment of traumatic intracranial mass lesions. It is practical yet based on a foundation of solid clinical and laboratory research. Most importantly, it draws on the extensive experience of two eminent authorities in the field who critically interpret the latest information and serve as wise guides in the management of this challenging group of patients.

Paul R. Cooper, MD
New York University Medical Center
New York, NY

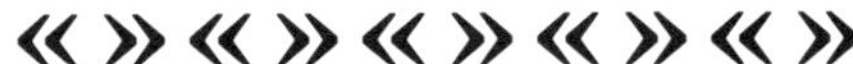

To our wives, Linda and Mary,
and our children, Lauren, Christopher,
Jennifer, and John

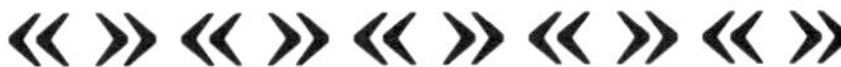

Preface

Head injury is a major public health problem in the United States, accounting for 44% of all deaths from trauma. Approximately 500,000 head injuries occur each year; 30% to 50% are at least moderately severe, 10% are fatal, and up to 10% of survivors suffer residual and often debilitating neurological deficits. Severe head trauma is most common in young adults 15–24 years of age, and males are four times as likely as females to sustain a fatal injury. Although the mechanisms vary somewhat by geographic region and patient age, motor vehicle accidents account for the majority of cases. Head injury is not only one of the most lethal and disabling health problems, but, by affecting a disproportionately large number of young persons, also deprives society of their productivity and results in a longstanding burden of care for handicapped survivors.

At our institution, a regional trauma center, as many as 10% of patients admitted with severe head injury have clinical signs of upper brain stem dysfunction consistent with transtentorial herniation. Although many of these patients may indeed have lethal parenchymal brain injuries, a significant number have treatable and potentially reversible brain stem compression. To maximize the potential for a successful outcome, this condition must be recognized promptly and treated without delay.

This monograph examines in detail the management of severe head injury, beginning with a review of the anatomy of the tentorial region and the pathophysiology and biomechanics of post-traumatic transtentorial herniation. Subsequent chapters are devoted to the neurological examination, initial resuscitation, radiographic assessment, critical care, and pharmacological therapy of severely head-injured patients. Although we have adopted an aggressive stance toward the diagnosis and treatment of transtentorial herniation, as discussed in chapters on burr-hole exploration and new methods of intraoperative brain imaging, we recognize that this approach remains controversial and acknowledge alternative methods or philosophies where appropriate. Our goal in writing this monograph is to emphasize the potential for a successful outcome in a subset of head-injured patients considered beyond hope by many clinicians.

Brian T. Andrews, MD
Lawrence H. Pitts, MD

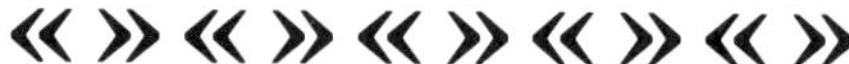

Acknowledgments

We would like to express our gratitude to the residents of the Department of Neurological Surgery, University of California, San Francisco, for their skill and dedication in caring for head-injured patients. We also thank Steven Korn of Futura Publishing Company for being so helpful in the development of this book. Finally, we are grateful to our editor, Stephen Ordway, for his invaluable collaboration.

Contents

CHAPTER 1

Anatomy, Biomechanics, and Pathology

The Tentorium Cerebelli

The tentorium cerebelli is an arched lamina of dura that lies in the cerebrocerebellar fissure. Formed of concentric, circumferential, and radial fibrous bands, it yields little to pressure[3] and has been described as a "mechanically perfect means of directing forces away from the vulnerable midbrain."[5] Elevated in the midline and slightly concave upward, the tentorium slopes downward, attaching to the petrous ridge laterally and to the transverse grooves of the occipital bone posteriorly (Fig. 1-1). The anteromedial border forms the concave edge of the incisura tentorii cerebelli, which converges with the attached margin of the tentorium at the petrous apex and continues forward to insert into the anterior and posterior clinoid processes; the posterior border is contiguous with the dura covering the transverse sinus.

The raised midline of the tentorium joins with the falx cerebri to form the straight sinus, which drains the vein of Galen. Along the petrous margin of the tentorium is formed the superior petrosal sinus, which drains the cavernous sinus; and along the occipital margin are formed the transverse or lateral sinuses, which drain the confluence of the straight sinus and superior and inferior sagittal sinuses at the torcular Herophili (Fig. 1-2).

In adults, the incisura tentorii cerebelli is approximately 25–35 mm in maximal width, 40–75 mm long,[4,5,20] and slopes upward about 40° from front to back; however, these dimensions vary

From *Traumatic Transtentorial Herniation and Its Management* by Brian T. Andrews, MD and Lawrence H. Pitts, MD © 1991, Futura Publishing Co., Inc., Mount Kisco, NY.

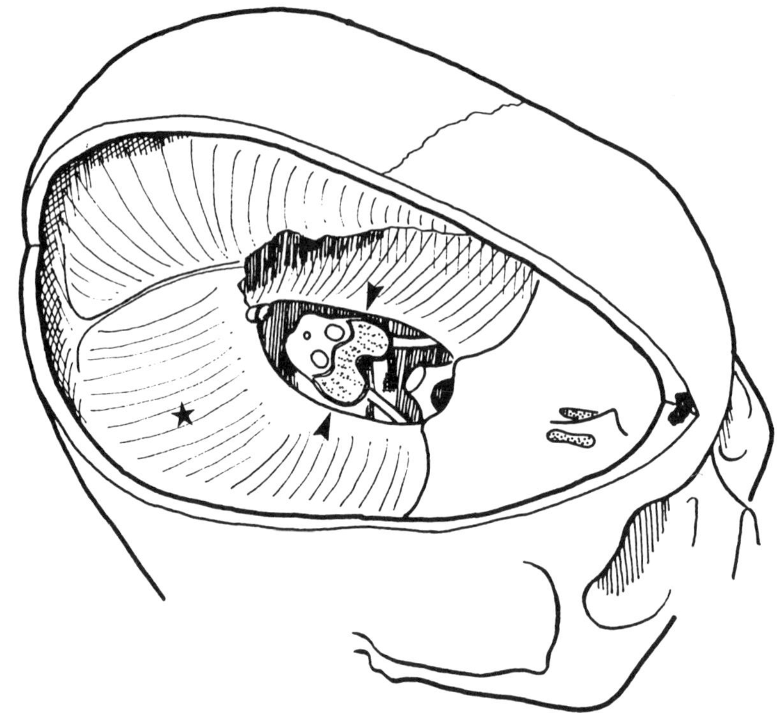

Figure 1-1. Overhead and angled right side views of the skull showing the tentorium *(star)* and the incisura *(arrowheads)* and their relationship to the midbrain and third cranial nerves.

considerably.[2,3] The incisura contains the cerebral peduncles, which average 30 mm in their widest dimension, the tegmentum, and the superior and inferior colliculi of the mesencephalon.[5] The space between the free edge of the tentorium and the mesencephalon varies; these structures touch in some cases and are separated by as much as 7 mm in others;[2,5,20] the lateral tentoriopeduncular space is absent in 43% of postmortem specimens.[5] The shape of the skull and the age of the patient may influence the size of the incisura and the amount of space between the mesencephalon and the lateral dural margins. The variability of these dimensions probably affects individual susceptibility to transtentorial herniation.

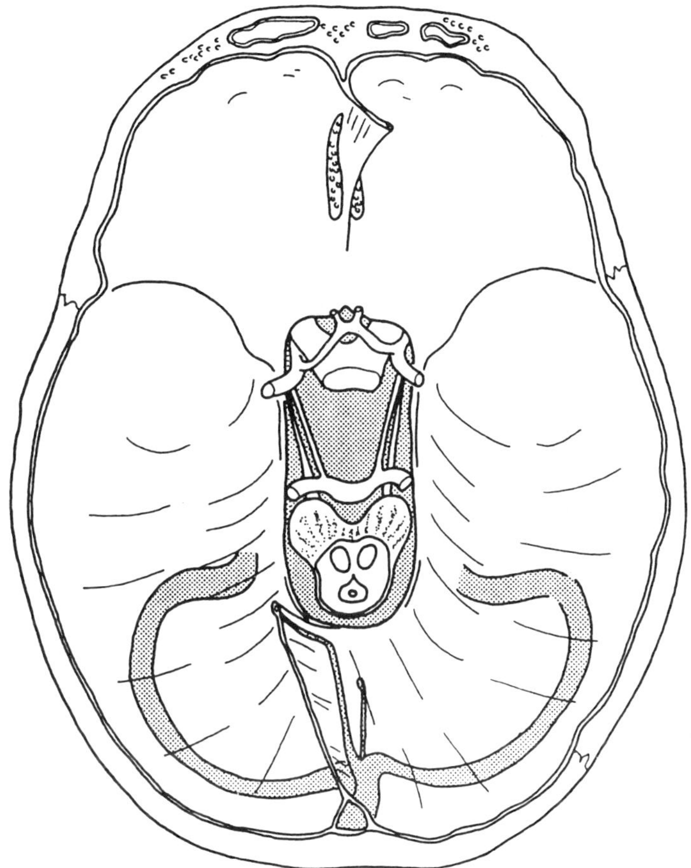

Figure 1-2. Overhead view of the tentorium. The straight and transverse sinuses are highlighted.

Structures within the Incisura

The third (oculomotor) cranial nerves emerge from a sulcus along the medial aspect of the cerebral peduncles, pass over the posterior clinoid processes, and enter the dura along the superior border of the cavernous sinuses (Fig. 1-3). The fibers of this nerve rotate 180° as they pass through the subarachnoid space.[13] The pupilloconstrictor fibers lie on the superior margin of the oculomotor nerve at the

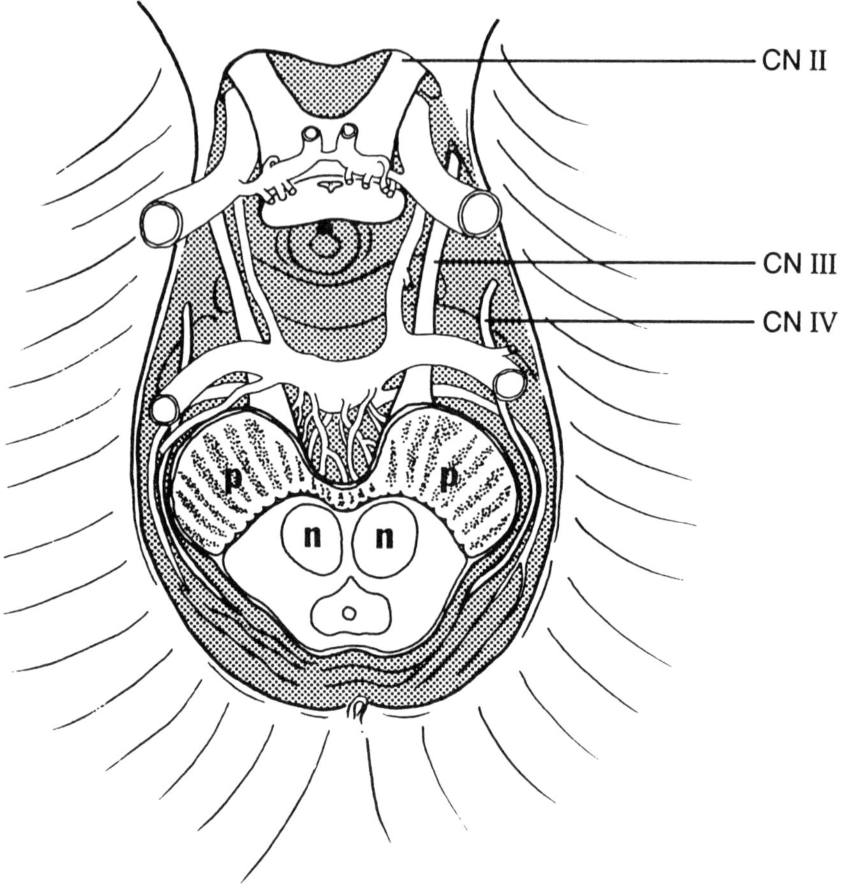

Figure 1-3. A more detailed overhead view of the contents of the tentorial incisura. The oculomotor nerves (CN III) from the cerebral peduncles (P) to the cavernous sinus, the adjacent arterial circle of Willis and their relationship to the midbrain and adjacent tentorial incisura are shown. The nuclei (n) of the oculomotor nerves are also shown. CN = cranial nerve.

cerebral peduncles and on the inferior margin as it enters the cavernous sinus.[21] These fibers are exquisitely sensitive to compression.[6,14] The medial margin of the uncus usually overhangs the incisura, and closely approximates each oculomotor nerve laterally.

Superior to the oculomotor nerves lie the posterior communicating arteries. These vessels arise anteriorly from the internal carotid arteries, run posteriorly, and cross the oculomotor nerves as the latter enter the dura of the cavernous sinus (Fig. 1-3). The posterior communicating arteries join with the posterior cerebral arteries, which arise from the distal bifurcation of the basilar artery and course laterally, crossing over the oculomotor nerves as they exit from the ventral brain stem. Inferior to the oculomotor nerves, the superior cerebellar arteries arise from the basilar trunk and run laterally under the tentorial margin.

The mesencephalon, or midbrain, consists of the cerebral peduncles anteriorly, the midportion or tegmentum, and the superior and inferior colliculi, or tectum, posteriorly (Fig. 1-3). All fiber tracts connecting the cerebral cortex, basal ganglia, thalamus, and the upper brain stem nuclei with the lower brain stem pass through the midbrain. Within this region lie the nuclei of the third and fourth cranial nerves, the substantia nigra, the red nuclei, the periaqueductal gray matter, and the pretectal nuclei, as well as critically important neuronal elements of the mesencephalic reticular activating system.

The blood supply to the midbrain consists primarily of the median perforating arteries, which branch from the terminal portion of the basilar artery in the interpeduncular fossa and from the origin of the posterior cerebral arteries at the ventral midbrain. The cerebral peduncles are largely supplied by the proximal posterior cerebral arteries.[5] These vessels give rise to the interpeduncular arteries, which supply the medial peduncles, and the oculomotor arteries, which enter the peduncles near the oculomotor nerves and supply midline structures anterior to the aqueduct of Sylvius, including the nuclei of the oculomotor nerves.

More inferiorly, smaller circumferential arteries arise transversely from the distal basilar artery and give off small arteries that penetrate the midbrain.[5] Median perforating branches also arising from the basilar artery and from the circumferential superior and anterior inferior cerebellar arteries irrigate the pons. These small perforating arteries supplying the upper brain stem are considered to be functional end arteries with few or no collaterals in the parenchyma; occlusion of one or several of these small vessels by mechanical compression usually causes severe ischemia in the upper brain stem.

Venous drainage of the midbrain and upper pons consists primarily of the prepontine venous plexus along the ventral midline of the pons and the basal vein of Rosenthal. These veins course antero-posteriorly around the mesencephalon within the ambient cistern and converge with the internal cerebral veins to form the great vein of Galen dorsal to the corpora quadrigemina.

The subarachnoid spaces surrounding the mesencephalon are divided into several paratentorial cisterns that protect the midbrain by acting as hydraulic buffers.[5] Anterior and medial to the cerebral peduncles lies the interpeduncular cistern; more caudally and ventral to the pons is the pontine cistern. Others have described the entire ventral space as the basal cistern.[5] Lateral to the mesencephalon lies the ambient cistern, or space of Bichat.[5] Posterior to the mesencephalon is the quadrigeminal plate cistern, which is also called the cistern of the great vein of Galen or the cisterna transversa.

Biomechanics and Pathology

The term *transtentorial herniation* describes the medial and caudal dislocation of brain parenchyma through the tentorial incisura.[5] Downward herniation occurs when one or both temporal lobes are forced down through the incisura and is the more common form. Upward herniation occurs when the superior cerebellar vermis is forced up through the incisura by a posterior fossa mass. In 1896, Hill demonstrated downward herniation in dogs by inflating a balloon in the supratentorial space.[7] Intracranial pressure increased most above the tentorium, less below the tentorium, and least in the spinal subarachnoid space. Hill concluded that displaced tissue within the tentorial notch and at the foramen magnum caused a tamponade, resulting in a pressure differential between the supra- and infratentorial compartments and the spinal canal.[7]

In 1939 Sorgo[18] injected paraffin into the parietal subdural space of cats. Autopsy showed herniation of brain tissue into the ipsilateral ambient cistern and compression of the third cranial nerve nucleus and the aqueduct of Sylvius. The next year, Perret[16] found that prior decompression of the posterior fossa resulted in more immediate herniation when a similar parietal mass was applied. In 1956 Cabieses[1] repeated these experiments in human cadavers and filmed the results. Initially, the brain stem was displaced caudally and contralaterally, and then the uncus and hippocampus herniated into the ambient cistern ipsilateral to the mass lesion.

In 1960 Jennett and Stern inflated extra-axial balloons in the supratentorial compartment of cats and monkeys to produce frontal, temporal, and bifrontal compressions.[10] These studies also showed mechanical distortion and downward impaction of the brain stem, which compressed the third cranial nerves.

Recently Zirski et al.[22] reported that an increase in intracranial pressure caused by inflation of a unilateral supratentorial extra-axial balloon in cats resulted in a decrease in regional cerebral blood flow in both cerebral hemispheres; the decrease occurred more rapidly ipsilateral to the mass lesion. Blood flow in the brain stem also decreased, but to a lesser extent. When balloon inflation was continued until transtentorial herniation developed, regional blood flow decreased much more in the upper brain stem than in the pons and medulla. This suggests that more pressure is transmitted to the upper brain stem than is directed more caudally.

These experimental studies provide evidence that a hemispheric mass lesion causes a brain shift, forcing the cerebral hemisphere across the edge of the tentorium into the incisura (Fig. 1-4).

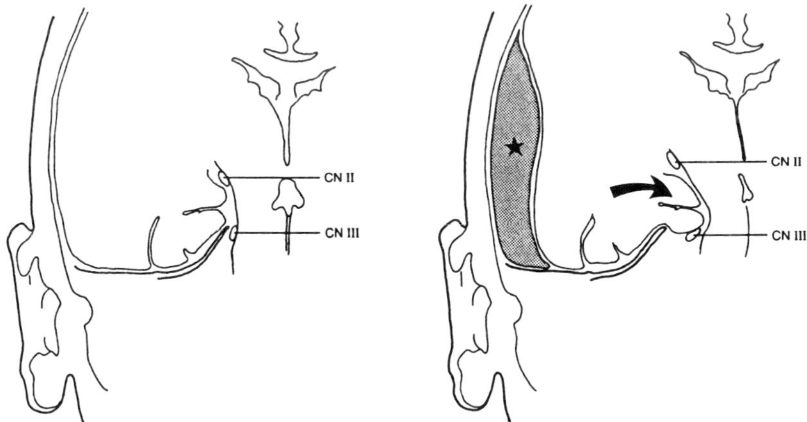

Figure 1-4. Diagram showing in a coronal plane the mechanism of transtentorial herniation caused by an expanding extra-axial hematoma *(star)*. Note the shifting of the medial temporal lobe and compression of the brain stem and cranial nerve III *(arrow)*.

Pressure is transmitted to the mesencephalon, and the entire brain stem is displaced caudally, which may result in further impactions of the medulla and the cerebellar tonsils at the foramen magnum. Regional blood flow decreases, especially to the upper brain stem.

Numerous studies of the pathology of transtentorial herniation in humans have confirmed these experimental findings. In 1920 Meyer[15] published a seminal photographic analysis of the major herniation syndromes of the brain. Transtentorial herniation caused medial deviation of the uncus, obliterated the ipsilateral ambient cistern, and compressed the midbrain, displacing it contralaterally. Jefferson[9] showed that the uncus alone could herniate anterior to the midbrain, whereas Johnson and Yates[11] showed that herniation of the lingual, fornicial, and cingulate gyri of the temporal lobe could occur more posteriorly.

Shallow grooves may be noted postmortem in the medial uncus of normal brain.[5,8,17] In transtentorial herniation, however, the firm edge of the tentorium causes a deep groove or notch in the undersurface of the ipsilateral uncus.[5,20] Severe herniation may compress and even occlude the aqueduct of Sylvius;[5,9] twist the brain stem, pushing it contralaterally; and elongate and flatten the ipsilateral cerebral peduncle. These deformations stretch the ipsilateral oculomotor nerve across the edge of the posterior clinoid process and slacken the contralateral third nerve.[5] The stalk of the pituitary gland may be stretched over the dorsum sella and cause pituitary infarction.[8] In some cases, progressive transtentorial herniation can result in the Kernohan's notch phenomenon, in which the displacement of the brain stem and diencephalic structures forces the contralateral crus of the cerebral peduncle against the contralateral edge of the tentorium (Fig. 1-5).[12]

In addition to temporal lobe herniation and deformation of the brain stem, transtentorial herniation causes severe distortion of the adjacent arteries of the posterior circulation. The small perforating arteries may be stretched and occluded by downward displacement of the brain stem or even rupture, resulting in hemorrhage within the tegmentum of the midbrain and pons (Duret's hemorrhages). The posterior cerebral arteries become stretched and compressed where they cross over the incisura and enter the supratentorial space.[5] Occlusion of these arteries and infarction of the occipital lobes are another complication of transtentorial herniation.

The herniated temporal lobe also undergoes the pathological

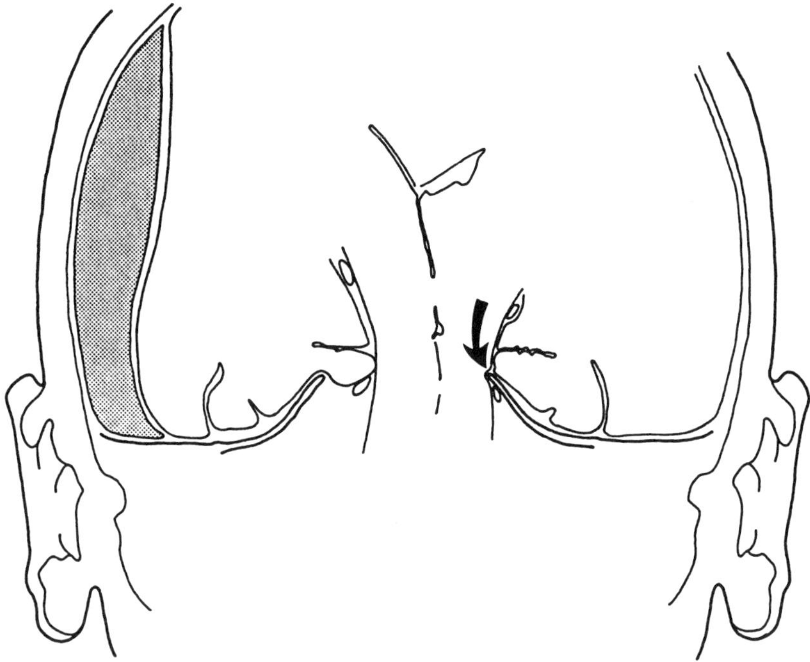

Figure 1-5. Diagram showing in a coronal plane the mechanism of transtentorial herniation that compresses the contralateral cerebral peduncle against the adjacent edge of the tentorium ("Kernohan's notch" phenomenon) *(arrow)*.

changes of lipid vacuolization and glial proliferation.[19] Neurons initially become swollen, and nuclei are peripherally displaced. In more chronic cases due to nontraumatic hemispheric mass lesions, the neurons become pyknotic, and fibrous gliosis develops. The brain stem becomes edematous, and changes similar to those associated with ischemia (pyknotic nuclei and poorly staining cytoplasm) occur in neurons of the brain stem ganglia. In cases of chronic transtentorial herniation caused by brain tumors, the cellular changes may be quite mild even when herniation proved fatal. Small hemorrhages resulting from vascular occlusion and small-vessel rupture may occur in the tegmentum of the midbrain and pons when these structures herniate downward.[8] Veins, venules, and capillaries in these regions may become dilated and thrombosed; these changes have been attributed to both ischemia and compression.[5]

Summary

Experimental and pathological data indicate that a unilateral hemispheric mass lesion of sufficient size causes a brain shift that forces the medial aspect of the temporal lobe at the uncus anteriorly or more posteriorly at the cingulate gyrus to herniate across the tentorial edge and into the incisura. Transmitted pressure compresses, twists, and displaces the entire brain stem contralaterally and caudally. The large arteries of the posterior circulation are displaced and distorted; the posterior cerebral artery is compressed and occluded, and the smaller perforating arteries supplying the brain stem are occluded as well. The ensuing severe decrease in blood flow to the upper brain stem and occipital lobes causes ischemic infarction. Injury to the small perforating vessels may also cause brain stem hemorrhage. The ipsilateral third cranial nerve may be stretched, and the cerebral peduncles may be compressed ipsilaterally or contralaterally (Kernohan's notch phenomenon).

References

1. Cabieses F: El Tronco Encefalico en las Lesiones Expansivas Supratentoriales. Lima, Peru: Universidad Nacional Major de San Marcos Facultad de Medicina, 1956, p 231.
2. Corsellis JAN: Individual variation in the size of the tentorial opening. J Neurol Neurosurg Psychiatry 21:279-283, 1958.
3. Dott NM: The brain and the skull. In: Thompson A, Miles A (eds.): Manual of Surgery. 9th ed. Oxford: Oxford Medical Publications, 1939, pp 663-695.
4. Echols DH, Rickles JA: Herniation of the temporal lobe into the cerebellar fossa. New Orleans Med Soc J 98:408-411, 1946.
5. Finney LA, Walker AE: Transtentorial Herniation. Springfield, IL: Charles C Thomas, 1962, pp 12-26.
6. Fisher CM: Oval pupils. Arch Neurol 37:502-503, 1980.
7. Hill L: The physiology and pathology of the cerebral circulation. London: J. and A. Churchill, 1896, p 208.

8. Howell DA: Upper brain stem compression and foraminal impaction with intracranial space–occupying lesions and brain swelling. Brain 82:525-550, 1959.
9. Jefferson G: Tentorial pressure cone. Arch Neurol Psychiatry 40:857-876, 1940.
10. Jennett WB, Stern WE: Tentorial herniation, the midbrain and the pupil. Experimental studies in brain compression. J Neurosurg 17:598-609, 1960.
11. Johnson RT, Yates PO: Clinico–pathological aspects of pressure changes at the tentorium. Acta Radiol 46:242, 1956.
12. Kernohan JW, Woltman HE: Incisura of the crus due to contralateral brain tumor. Arch Neurol Psychiatry 21:274-287, 1929.
13. Lazorthes G, Gaubert J, Planel H: Le trajet des fibres de la motricité intrinsèque dans le III nerf cranien. A. des Anatomistes 41:473-477, 1954.
14. Marshall LF, Barba D, Toole BM, et al.: The oval pupil: clinical significance and relationship to intracranial hypertension. J Neurosurg 58:566-568, 1983.
15. Meyer A: Herniation of the brain. Arch Neurol Psychiatry 4: 387-400, 1920.
16. Perret GE: Experimentelle Untersuchung über Massenverschiebungen und Formveranderungen des Gehirns bei raumbeengenden Prozessen. Zentralbl Neurochir 5:5-29, 1940.
17. Schwartz GA, Rosner AA: Displacement and herniation of hippocampal gyrus through the incisura tentorii: a clinicopathological study. Arch Neurol Psychiatry 46:297-321, 1941.
18. Sorgo W: Experimentelle Untersuchungen über die Klinik der Verquellung der Cisterna ambiens. Dtsch Z Nervenh 149:271-283, 1939.
19. Spatz H, Stroescu GJ: Zur Anatomie und Pathologie der ausseren Liquorraume des Gehrins. Nervenarzt 7:481-498, 1934.
20. Sunderland S: The tentorial notch and complications produced by herniations of brain through that aperture. Br J Surg 45:422-438, 1958.
21. Sunderland S, Hughes ESR: The pupilloconstrictor pathway and the nerves to the ocular muscles in man. Brain 69:301-309, 1946.
22. Zierski J, Kurzaj E, Hoffman O, et al.: Cerebral blood flow in the brain stem during increased intracranial pressure. In: Ishii S, Nagai H, Brock M (eds): Intracranial Pressure V. Berlin: Springer-Verlag Publishers, 1983, pp 452-455.

CHAPTER 2

Clinical Manifestations

Upper brain stem compression due to herniation of the uncus across the edge of the tentorium causes a classic triad of clinical signs: a depressed level of consciousness, anisocoria with ipsilateral pupillary dilatation and loss of the light reflex, and an abnormal motor response.[5] It is critically important to recognize this triad in severely head-injured patients and to realize that the clinical signs usually evolve. Often, deterioration to coma follows a so-called lucid period. In some cases, one pupil may be dilated but reactive initially; but as brain stem compression worsens, both pupils may become dilated and unreactive. Similarly, in the earliest stages of herniation, a hemiparesis may not be detectable; but as hemispheric and brain stem compression increase, the motor response worsens, and an asymmetrical, usually contralateral, hemiparesis may develop, followed by further progression to quadriparesis or bilateral flaccidity. In such cases, *ongoing* deterioration of these clinical signs almost invariably reflects an expanding intracranial mass lesion, which must be recognized to allow timely intervention and appropriate management.

Neuroanatomical Basis of Clinical Signs

In 1939 Sorgo[9] found that transtentorial herniation induced by injecting paraffin into the parietal subdural space of cats initially caused a decrease in the ipsilateral direct light reflex, which was followed by the onset of ipsilateral pupillary dilatation. He believed these findings indicated compression of the ipsilateral third cranial nerve nucleus rather than of the third nerve itself. Tarlov and

From *Traumatic Transtentorial Herniation and Its Management* by Brian T. Andrews, MD and Lawrence H. Pitts, MD © 1991, Futura Publishing Co., Inc., Mount Kisco, NY.

Giancotti[10] studied the clinical effects of experimental transtentorial herniation in dogs and detected progressive impairment of consciousness, ipsilateral pupillary constriction, and decerebrate rigidity. Respiration slowed with the onset of bradycardia, but hypertension did not occur uniformly. Jennet and Stern[2] produced transtentorial herniation similar to that seen in man by inflating intracranial balloons in the supratentorial space in monkeys. Bifrontal compression caused bilateral pupillary dilatation and decreased the respiratory rate; unilateral compression most often resulted in unilateral pupillary dilatation. Electrical stimulation testing showed that the pupillary changes resulted from a direct effect of herniation on the nerve.

Level of Consciousness

In humans, the level of consciousness reflects both the level of arousal and the presence of cognition or conscious behavior. Arousal is dependent upon proper function of the reticular activating system (RAS), whereas conscious behavior is dependent upon proper function of the cortical hemispheres.[7] Alterations in the level of consciousness in transtentorial herniation may result either from compression of the midbrain that disrupts function of the RAS or from the effect of the traumatic injury or the intracranial mass lesion on neocortical function.

The RAS is a diffuse network of neurons in the brain stem. Most prominent in the midbrain, where it forms a part of the tegmentum, it also extends into the subthalamus and hypothalamus of the diencephalon. Although its borders are indistinct, the RAS contains a number of discrete nuclei. The neurons of the RAS are extensively interconnected and receive collateral input from every major somatic and special sensory pathway, particularly the spinothalamic system and the trigeminal nerve. Numerous axons from the RAS ascend through the central tegmental fasciculus of the midbrain and extend into the thalamus, the hypothalamus, the basal forebrain structures, including the limbic system, and diffusely into the neocortex.[7] There is also extensive reciprocal innervation from each of these cortical and subcortical structures back into the RAS.

Stimulation of the RAS produces a generalized nonspecific activation of the cerebral cortex. This appears to occur in part through abolition of the tonically inhibitory influence of the thalamic reticular nucleus and through modulation of the limbic system by the hypothalamus. An injury that interrupts or reduces rostral input from the RAS in the mesencephalon and diencephalon decreases alertness and cortical arousal. In transtentorial herniation, such injury occurs as a result of compression or ischemia in the midbrain.

Conscious behavior is dependent upon arousal of the cerebral cortex in many localized areas that participate in specific cognitive functions. Of special importance are sensory and sensory association areas and regions important for motivation, such as the frontal cortex, and memory, including the temporal cortex. Conscious behavior may also be disproportionately linked to the function of language-producing areas of the dominant hemisphere.[7]

Cortical lesions of increasing size cause a progressive decrease in alertness and cognitive function, regardless of their location. When cortical function ceases, the patient loses all alertness, even if the RAS remains intact.[1] Damage to connections between cortical regions probably explains the influence of a lesion on uninjured areas. Intact cognitive function may require continuous afferent stimulation from all other parts of the neocortex through both corticothalamic and direct cortical connections.[7]

Pupillary Function

Pupillary size and reactivity are determined by the balance between the effects of the sympathetic and parasympathetic nervous systems on the pupils. Sympathetic innervation arises from the hypothalamus and brain stem, passing through the cervical spinal cord to synapses in the intermediolateral tract of the upper three thoracic spinal segments. Preganglionic fibers pass through the ventral roots of the cervical spinal cord and through the inferior and middle cervical sympathetic ganglia to synapses in the superior cervical sympathetic ganglion. Postganglionic fibers pass through the internal carotid plexus along the internal carotid artery, enter the orbit through the superior orbital fissure with the nasociliary nerve, and then enter the globe as the long ciliary nerve. Sympathetic discharges innervate the dilator pupillae muscle, resulting in dilatation of the pupil. Sympathetic fibers also innervate the smooth muscle of the levators of the eyelid (Mueller's muscle).

Parasympathetic innervation arises from the Edinger-Westphal nucleus, dorsal to the third nerve nucleus in the mesencephalon. The preganglionic fibers travel with the oculomotor nerve as it passes forward from the interpeduncular fossa and pierces the dural edge of the incisura to enter the lateral wall of the cavernous sinus. The parasympathetic fibers lie peripherally in the nerve and are exquisitely sensitive to compression. Where the oculomotor nerve enters the superior orbital fissure, the parasympathetic fibers travel to the ciliary ganglion and synapse. The postganglionic fibers form the short ciliary nerve, which enters the sclera and innervates the smooth muscle fibers that constrict the pupil.

Transtentorial herniation affects pupillary function by compressing either the ipsilateral third nerve nucleus and the Edinger-Westphal nucleus or the oculomotor nerve itself (see Chapter 1, Fig. 1-4). Even relatively mild increases in intracranial pressure may cause pupillary dilation or irregularity, probably as a result of compression or torsion of these fibers along their rather long intracranial course.[4] Compression of the nerve may result first in the loss of parasympathetic tone; with continued sympathetic innervation, the ipsilateral pupil becomes enlarged and sometimes irregular (Fig. 2-1).[4] Selhorst et al.[8] suggest that an oval or irregular pupil may

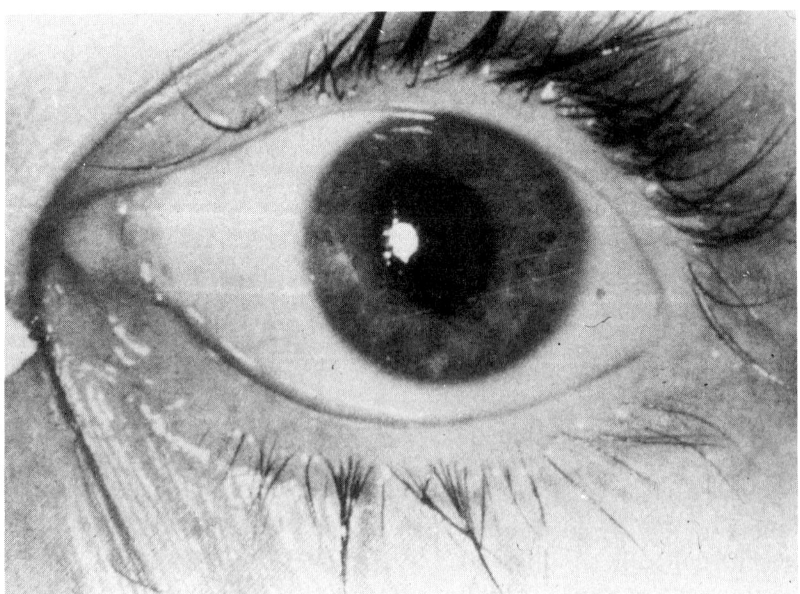

Figure 2-1. An enlarged and irregular pupil caused by transtentorial herniation that compresses the ipsilateral oculomotor nerve (CN III).

result from centrally determined differences in parasympathetic tone to some segments of the pupillary sphincters. As transtentorial herniation progresses, causing compression and probably ischemia of the midbrain, both parasympathetic and sympathetic innervation may be lost, resulting in midposition (4–5 mm) pupils that do not react (i.e., are "fixed") to light. If transtentorial herniation persists and the more central fibers of the oculomotor nerve supplying the extraocular muscles are affected, third-nerve-mediated ipsilateral extraocular movements may be lost.

Hemiparesis

Asymmetrical motor findings, the third component of the classic triad, consist most often of a contralateral hemiparesis, which is usually attributed to uncal compression on the corticospinal tracts in the ventrolateral aspect of the ipsilateral cerebral peduncle (see Chapter 1, Fig. 1-4). However, compression or primary injury in the motor region of the cortical hemisphere itself, above the cerebral peduncle,[6] may also cause contralateral hemiparesis. In approximately 25% of cases, the hemiparesis is ipsilateral to the dilated pupil[6] because the brain stem is displaced away from the side of the mass, compressing the contralateral cerebral peduncle against the opposite dural edge of the incisura (see Chapter 1, Fig. 1-5) (Kernohan's notch phenomenon).[3]

References

1. Dougherty JH Jr, Rawlinson D, Levy DE, et al.: Hypoxic ischemic brain injury and the vegetative state: clinical and neuropathological correlation. Neurology 29:591, 1979
2. Jennett WB, Stern WE: Tentorial herniation, the midbrain and the pupil. Experimental studies in brain compression. J Neurosurg 17:598-609, 1960.
3. Kernohan JW, Woltman HE: Incisura of the crus due to contralateral brain tumor. Arch Neurol Psychiatry 21:274-287, 1929.
4. Marshall LF, Barba D, Toole BM, et al.: The oval pupil: clinical significance and relationship to intracranial hypertension. J Neurosurg 58:566-568, 1983.

5. Meyer A: Herniation of the brain. Arch Neurol Psychiatry 4: 387-400, 1920.
6. Pitts LH: Neurological evaluation of the head injury patient. Clin Neurosurg 29:203-224, 1981.
7. Plum F, Posner JB: The Diagnosis of Stupor and Coma. 3rd ed. Philadelphia: FA Davis Publishers, 1980, pp 1-86.
8. Selhorst JB, Hoyt WF, Feinsod M: Midbrain corectopia. Arch Neurol 33:193-195, 1976.
9. Sorgo W: Experimentelle Untersuchungen über die Klinik der Verquellung der Cisterna ambiens. Dtsch Z Nervenh 149:271-283, 1939.
10. Tarlov IM, Gianocotti A: Acute increased intracranial pressure: an experimental clinical study aiding diagnosis. Trans Am Neurol Assoc 81:118-124, 1956.

CHAPTER 3

Initial Assessment

Despite the increasing use of sophisticated diagnostic and monitoring techniques, the clinical examination remains the simplest, most reliable, and most important tool for evaluating severely head-injured patients.[17] Each component of the initial examination is important. The admission history and physical examination may yield information on the mechanism of injury, injuries to other parts of the body, concurrent medical conditions, and complicating features, such as drug intoxication, that may mask the true extent of neurological damage. The neurological examination provides baseline data upon which initial management decisions are based[2,14,18] and upon which the neurological outcome may rest.[3,4,6–9,11,12,14,15,19] The ability to assess the clinical status of the patient quickly and accurately and to record the findings in a standardized fashion for comparison with subsequent findings is crucial in managing head-injured patients.

At San Francisco General Hospital Medical Center, all patients with suspected severe head injury are evaluated upon arrival in the emergency room by a trauma team that includes members of the neurosurgical and general (trauma) surgical services and, if necessary, other services such as orthopedics, urology, and ophthalmology. A designated member of the surgical team directs and coordinates the initial evaluation and ensures that resuscitation proceeds while the extent of systemic injuries is being established and a neurological evaluation is performed.

From *Traumatic Transtentorial Herniation and Its Management* by Brian T. Andrews, MD and Lawrence H. Pitts, MD © 1991, Futura Publishing Co., Inc., Mount Kisco, NY.

Admission History

It is imperative that some effort be made to determine the circumstances surrounding the accident. The admission history may be reported by witnesses to the accident or by paramedics based on their findings at the scene. Information from these sources or from family members may provide clues to factors that influence the physical and neurological findings. The sudden onset of a headache, seizure, or loss of consciousness before the accident, for example, might suggest an underlying condition, such as acute subarachnoid or intraparenchymal hemorrhage or myocardial infarction. There may be evidence of drug use or ethanol intoxication, which depresses neurological function.[10,17] The type of accident may suggest specific additional injuries. Impact against the steering wheel may cause pulmonary or cardiac contusions and lead to systemic hypoxia or hypotension, either of which may depress neurological function.[1] A cervical spinal cord injury resulting from a diving accident or impact against a windshield might drastically alter the neurological findings. The time of injury may also prove useful. If there has been a prolonged delay before the patient is brought to the emergency room, the effects of hemorrhagic hypotension or systemic hypoxia due to pulmonary hypoventilation may exacerbate the neurological insult of the head injury.

Physical and Neurological Examinations

The neurological findings are recorded on a standardized form (Fig. 3-1) to document them for comparison with subsequent findings and to help prevent errors of omission during the evaluation. As the neurological examination proceeds, the examiner must be aware of the presence of systemic injuries and the stability of the vital signs, including heart rate, blood pressure, and respiratory rate. Severe systemic hypotension[1] or hypoxia[14,17] must be identified and corrected as promptly and completely as possible because either may cause abnormal neurological findings due to cerebral ischemia; the vital signs and pulmonary function must be closely monitored for the delayed development of systemic hypotension. Arterial blood gases should be measured to evaluate oxygenation and to determine if metabolic acidosis is present. A urine sample should be obtained

DATE TIME	PROBLEM NUMBER	FORMAT: PROBLEM NUMBER AND TITLE: S—Subjective A—Analysis O—Objective P—Plans
		NEUROSURGICAL HEAD INJURY ADMITTING SHEET
		Sex: ☐ Male / ☐ Female Age: Handedness: ☐ Left / ☐ Right
		Cause of Injury:
		Time from: Injury → Coma Injury → MEH Injury → Neuro Consult
	Physical Exam	Vital Signs BP HR TEMP

COMA SCORE	GROUP A	GROUP B	GROUP C	GROUP D
Eye Opening	None		To Pain	To Voice Spontaneously
Verbal Response	None	Sounds	Words	Confused Oriented
Motor Response	None Abnl. Extens. Abnl. Flexs.	Withdraws Localizes Pain		Follows Commands
	ALL circles here = A	HIGHEST circle here = B	ANY circle here = C	ALL circles must be here to = D

MOTOR EXAM:

	R	L
arms		
legs		

1 = no response
2 = abnormal extension
3 = abnormal flexion
4 = weakness
5 = normal

Spontaneous spasms (posturing)? ☐ Yes / ☐ No

PUPILS:	Ⓡ Size____mm Reaction + / - Ⓛ Size____mm Reaction + / -
EOMs:	III nerve palsy? ☐ Right ☐ Left ☐ Neither ☐ Both
	Spontaneous eye movements? Describe:
	Doll's eyes: ☐ Absent ☐ Sluggish ☐ Brisk ☐ Normal (awake)
	Calorics: ☐ None ☐ Dysconj. ☐ Conj. ☐ Nystagmus (BEST RESPONSE EITHER EAR)
CORNEALS:	Right + / - Left + / -
RESPIRATIONS:	☐ Regular ☐ Ataxic ☐ Periodic (Cheyne-Stokes)
	Apneic? ☐ Yes ☐ No Resp. Rate:
	Cough? ☐ Yes ☐ No Gag? ☐ Yes ☐ No

F 726N Rev. 8/87

Figure 3-1. The neurological admission form used at San Francisco General Hospital Medical Center.

to screen for alcohol, opiates, barbiturates, benzodiazepine, or other drugs that affect neurological function.[17] Serum electrolytes, blood urea nitrogen, creatinine, and liver function tests are also measured, because an abnormality in any of them may worsen abnormalities of neurological function;[16] serum osmolality will be elevated in patients with dehydration, alcohol intoxication, or hyperglycemia. Hypothermia, especially a core body temperature below 29° C, may also depress neurological function;[16] therefore, the neurological examination must be repeated as the patient is being rewarmed. Although important, detecting and treating metabolic and physical abnormalities *must not delay the search for correctable intracranial lesions.*

Injuries to the cervical vertebrae and ligaments may affect the sensory and motor functions of the extremities and limit the accuracy of the neurological evaluation of those areas. Therefore, a lateral radiograph of the cervical spine should be obtained with a portable x-ray machine as soon as possible. Until the results of the radiographic study are known, the neck should be kept immobilized in the neutral position on a spine board by taping across the forehead and placing sandbags on either side without axial traction[5] (Fig. 3-2). One must bear in mind that a single lateral cervical radiograph may not show significant cervical spinal injury in up to 20% of patients; even a more complete study, including anteroposterior and open-mouth odontoid views, may fail to show an injury in up to 8% of patients.[13] If a cervical injury is identified, the neck should remain immobilized until computerized tomography scans or other studies can be performed or until the patient is placed in cervical traction using Gardner-Wells or halo pin fixation of the skull.

Although a full examination may be deferred until the patient is stabilized, the thoracic and lumbar spine should be inspected and palpated early in the examination. Areas of tenderness, swelling, ecchymoses, or palpable abnormalities should be further evaluated

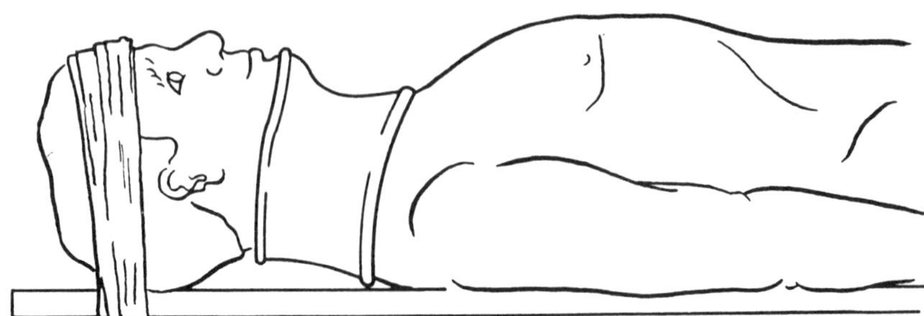

Figure 3-2. Tape securing the cervical spine of a patient immobilized on a firm back board.

with appropriate radiographs. An anteroposterior radiograph of the chest should also be obtained because of the potential for associated chest or pulmonary injury. If it shows widening of the mediastinum, a lower cervical or upper thoracic spinal fracture must be ruled out with additional studies, even if spinal cord function appears to be intact.[21]

External evidence of head trauma should be noted, including scalp lacerations and contusions, subgaleal hematomas, and deformities of the skull suggesting depressed skull fractures. If signs of basilar skull fracture, including periorbital ecchymoses, hemotympanum, and retroauricular ecchymoses (Battle's sign), are present, evidence of a cerebrospinal fluid leak should be sought. Ocular trauma must be ruled out because pupillary abnormalities, such as anisocoria or loss of reactivity, can result from injury to the globe rather than from intracranial compression of the third nerve.

Detailed tests of sensation, visual fields, and higher cortical function may not be possible in comatose or lethargic patients. Nonetheless, the examiner must accurately assess the status of hemispheric and brain stem function. The best way to assess hemispheric function is the Glasgow coma score (GCS) (Table 3-1).[19] The GCS reliably measures the level of consciousness, is easy to use, is repro-

Table 3-1. Glasgow Coma Scale

Category	*Response*	*Score*
Eye opening		
	None	1
	To pain	2
	To voice	3
	Spontaneously	4
Verbal		
	None	1
	Incomprehensible	2
	Garbled words	3
	Confused speech	4
	Oriented speech	5
Motor		
	Flaccid	1
	Abnormal extension	2
	Abnormal flexion	3
	Normal flexion	4
	Localizing pain	5
	Follows commands	6

ducible between examiners, and has powerful prognostic value as a measure of the severity of brain injury.[11] The GCS should be determined as a part of the initial examination and monitored repeatedly during subsequent management.

Brain stem function should be evaluated by testing brain stem reflexes. Pupillary reactivity and symmetry reflect the integrity of the midbrain, including the third nerve nuclei and superior colliculi, and the exiting third cranial nerves. The corneal reflexes reflect the integrity of the fifth and seventh cranial nerves and their interconnections in the pons. If cervical spinal injury has been ruled out, the oculocephalic reflex (doll's eye maneuver) should be examined to assess the midbrain and pons, specifically the integrity of the median longitudinal fasciculus. The oculovestibular reflex may be evaluated by the cold water caloric test as an additional assessment of the function of the pons and its connections to the midbrain. The gag and cough reflexes must be examined to evaluate medullary function. Finally the patient's respiratory status should be checked to assess the pontomedullary respiration centers.

A massive brain injury may cause apnea at admission to the emergency room. Apnea in combination with complete loss of cortical hemispheric function and the absence of all other brain stem reflexes may indicate that the patient is brain dead.[16] However, declaration of brain death requires a careful exclusion of reversible conditions, such as hypoxia or hypotension, drug intoxication, metabolic abnormalities, and hypothermia (see Chapter 13). On rare occasions when obvious and massive brain injury is readily apparent and reversible conditions have been evaluated and corrected without recovery of cortical or brain stem function, a declaration of brain death can be made at the initial evaluation using the guidelines summarized in Chapter 13.

References

1. Andrews BT, Levy ML, Pitts LH: The implication of systemic hypotension for the neurological examination in patients with severe head injury. Surg Neurol 28:419-422, 1987.
2. Andrews BT, Pitts LH, Lovely MP, et al.: Is computed tomographic scanning necessary in patients with tentorial herniation? Results of immediate surgical exploration without computed tomography in 100 patients. Neurosurgery 19:408-413, 1986.

3. Becker DP, Miller JD, Ward JD, et al.: The outcome from severe head injury with early diagnosis and intensive management. J Neurosurg 47:491-502, 1977.
4. Berger MS, Pitts LH, Lovely MP, et al.: Outcome from severe head injury in children and adolescents. J Neurosurg 62:194-199, 1985.
5. Bivins HG, Ford S, Bezmalinovic Z, et al.: The effect of axial traction during orotracheal intubation of the trauma victim with an unstable cervical spine. Ann Emerg Med 17:25-29, 1988.
6. Bowers SA, Marshall LF: Outcome in 200 consecutive cases of severe head injury treated in San Diego County: a prospective analysis. Neurosurgery 6:237-241, 1980.
7. Bricolo A, Turazzi S, Alexandre A, et al.: Decerebrate rigidity in acute head injury. J Neurosurg 47:680-696, 1977.
8. Bruce DA, Schut L, Bruno LA, et al.: Outcome following severe head injuries in children. J Neurosurg 48:679-688, 1978.
9. Gutterman P, Shenkin HA: Prognostic features in recovery from traumatic tentorial decerebration. J Neurosurg 32:330-335, 1970.
10. Jager J, Fife D, Vernberg K, et al.: Effect of alcohol intoxication on the diagnosis and apparent severity of brain injury. Neurosurgery 15:303-306, 1984.
11. Jennett B, Teasdale G, Braakman R, et al.: Prognosis of patients with severe head injury. Neurosurgery 4:283-288, 1979.
12. Lokkeberg AR, Grimes RM: Assessing the influence of non-treatment variables in a study of outcome from severe head injury. J Neurosurg 61:254-262, 1984.
13. Mace SE: Emergency evaluation of cervical spine injuries: CT versus plain radiographs. Ann Emerg Med 14:973-975, 1985.
14. Miller JD, Sweet RC, Narayan R, et al.: Early insults to the injured brain. JAMA 240:439-442, 1978.
15. Overgaard J, Hvid-Hansen O, Land AM, et al.: Prognosis after head injury based on early clinical examination. Lancet 2:631-635, 1973.
16. Pitts LH: Determination of brain death. West J Med 140:628-631, 1984.
17. Pitts LH: Neurological evaluation of the head injury patient. Clin Neurosurg 29:203-224, 1981.
18. Stone JL, Rifai R, Sugar KO, et al.: Subdural hematomas. I. Acute subdural hematoma: progress in definition, clinical pathology and therapy. Surg Neurol 19:216-231, 1983.

19. Teasdale G, Jennett B: Assessment of coma and impaired consciousness: a practical scale. Lancet 2:81-84, 1974.
20. Williams JM, Gomes F, Drudge OW, et al.: Predicting outcome from closed head injury by early assessment of trauma severity. J Neurosurg 61:581-585, 1984.
21. Woodring JH, Lee C, Jenkins K: Spinal fractures in blunt chest trauma. J Trauma 28:789-793, 1988.

CHAPTER 4

Resuscitation and Early Management

Treatment of severe head injury must be undertaken while the initial physical and neurological examinations and diagnostic studies are being performed. Thus, it must be assumed that there is a severe head injury before that fact has been established and before it is known if severe hypoxia, hypothermia, or drug intoxication has affected neurological function. Treatment is initiated based on clear evidence or a highly suggestive history of head injury in an apparently comatose patient.

Initially, all severe head injuries are managed the same way, regardless of whether clinical signs of transtentorial herniation are present. The immediate goals are to reduce elevated intracranial pressure (ICP), maintain effective cerebral oxygenation and perfusion, and prevent hypercarbia and acidosis. Cerebral perfusion pressure, defined as the mean arterial pressure minus the ICP, is normally about 80–90 mm Hg and must be at least 40 mm Hg to maintain adequate cerebral blood flow in the normal brain.[31] Thus, supporting the mean arterial blood pressure and lowering elevated ICP are essential to maintain adequate perfusion pressure. Hyperventilation and intravenous (IV) mannitol infusion are the primary means of achieving those goals and may also allow the brain to accommodate temporarily an underlying cause of increased ICP, such as an intracranial mass lesion, until it can be identified and treated directly. In patients with clinical signs of transtentorial her-

From *Traumatic Transtentorial Herniation and Its Management* by Brian T. Andrews, MD and Lawrence H. Pitts, MD © 1991, Futura Publishing Co., Inc., Mount Kisco, NY.

niation, extra-axial mass lesions are frequently the cause of increased ICP and brain stem compression.[1,35] Therefore early treatment with hyperventilation and mannitol are potentially even more crucial than in other severely head-injured patients.

At San Francisco General Hospital, the impending arrival of a patient with an apparent severe head injury is reported by radio from the accident scene. A multispecialty trauma team that includes an anesthesiologist, a trauma surgeon, and a neurosurgeon is quickly assembled in the emergency room, and preparations are made to evaluate neurological and systemic injuries and resuscitate the patient. The initial assessment by the members of this team has already been described (see Chapter 2).

Initial Resuscitation: The ABCs

The initial steps to resuscitate the severely head-injured patient are the same as for any trauma patient with significant injuries: to confirm that the patient has an airway, is breathing, and has adequate circulation (Fig. 4-1, Table 4-1). Upon arrival at the scene of the accident, paramedics attempt to establish an airway, usually by placing an oral airway and administering supplemental oxygen by mask. The use of an esophageal obturator airway in the field[30] has been criticized[29] and is not recommended. An IV line is usually

Table 4-1 Initial Resuscitation After Severe Head Injury: The ABCs
Airway
Initial mask ventilation with 100% oxygen
Endotracheal intubation if necessary and if no cervical spinal injuries are present
Breathing
Hyperventilation with 100% oxygen to maintain $Paco_2$ of 20–25 mm Hg and Po_2 greater than 100 mm Hg
Circulation
Establish adequate peripheral intravenous access (one or two 18-gauge intravenous catheters)
Intravenous infusion of lactated Ringer's solution (up to 2,000 ml) *if systolic blood pressure is < 80 mm Hg*
Transfusion of cross-matched or type-specific blood *for massive blood loss or for persistently low blood pressure*

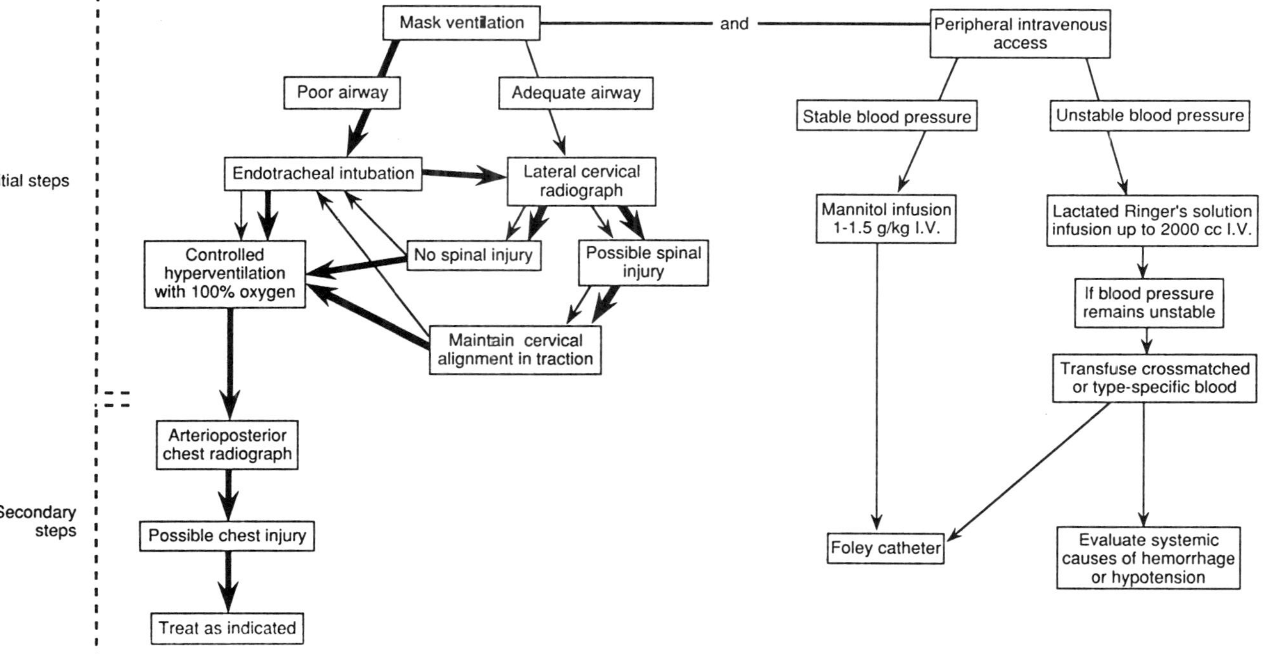

Figure 4-1. Flow chart showing the elements of the initial resuscitation and management of patients with transtentorial herniation. Bold arrows indicate steps taken in patients with a poor airway by mask ventilation. These patients must be intubated for controlled hyperventilation; a lateral cervical spinal x-ray is obtained simultaneously. Light arrows indicate steps in the management of patients with an adequate airway.

placed, and a crystalloid solution is infused. Cardiopulmonary resuscitation is performed if the patient is in cardiac arrest or has severe arterial hypotension.

Establishing an Airway

In the emergency room, the first step is to establish a patent airway. Initially, mask ventilation at a rapid ventilatory rate should be continued while a lateral cervical radiograph is quickly obtained. If there is no radiographic evidence of cervical spinal fractures or instability, standard orotracheal intubation may be used; extension of the cervical spine should still be avoided because there is a 20% chance of cervical injury despite a normal lateral radiograph.[33] If the airway cannot be maintained by mask ventilation, intubation must proceed immediately[15] using a technique that assumes that a spinal cord injury may be present. Orotracheal intubation may be performed with the head in the neutral position. Although it has been recommended,[9] gentle axial traction during orotracheal intubation may result in distraction of unstable spinal segments, especially in the upper cervical region, and should be avoided.[4] Alternatively, nasotracheal intubation or cricothyroidotomy may be performed;[2,4] however, if a major disruption of the skull base is suspected, blind nasotracheal intubation may be contraindicated because of the potential for intracranial passage of the tube.[10] Use of a fiberoptic laryngoscope may allow nasotracheal intubation under direct vision.[32]

Despite these cautions to prevent possible cervical injury, the incidence of *combined* head and spinal cord injuries is less than 5%.[20] The need for proper ventilation is so crucial that after the above techniques have been tried, more aggressive attempts to intubate the patient are appropriate to ensure an adequate airway.

Hyperventilation

Once an endotracheal tube has been inserted, hyperventilation with 100% oxygen should be started immediately to reduce elevated ICP.[16] By decreasing arterial carbon dioxide tension ($PaCO_2$), which increases the pH of blood and extracellular fluids,[12,13] hyperventilation induces a respiratory alkalosis. This in turn causes cerebral vasoconstriction,[12,13] which decreases cerebral blood volume, thereby reducing the volume of the brain and lowering the ICP, although not to the same degree in all patients.[21] Cerebral vasoconstriction increases as the $PaCO_2$ drops to 22–25 mm Hg; further decreases in $PaCO_2$ generally do not result in further vasoconstriction[21,24] and should be avoided to prevent metabolic complications from excessive alkalosis. A $PaCO_2$ less than 20 mm Hg may reduce cerebral blood flow below the level required for normal metabolism.[11] The vasoconstriction induced by hyperventilation is effective only in areas of the brain where CO_2 responsiveness is intact. Therefore, ICP may respond less to hyperventilation in patients with diffuse brain injuries and loss of cerebral CO_2 responsiveness than in those with more focal abnormalities or injury primarily to the brain stem,[21] in whom large regions of brain can still respond to hyperventilation.

Hypoxia and hypoventilation from injury to the lungs or chest are common among severely head-injured patients. Immediate hyperventilation with 100% oxygen can quickly reverse the effects of these pulmonary conditions, both of which may result in cerebral vasodilatation and thereby increase ICP. The respiratory alkalosis induced by hyperventilation tends, in addition, to reduce detrimental intracerebral acidosis.

Injuries to the chest and lungs that may inhibit adequate ventilation must be diagnosed and treated. Penetrating chest trauma can lead to both pulmonary and cardiac injury and potentially fatal hemorrhage, which may necessitate thoracotomy in the emergency room.[3] Blunt chest trauma can cause rib fractures, a flail segment of the chest, or pulmonary contusions, which may lead to pulmonary insufficiency; such injuries are best treated with intubation and positive pressure ventilation.[30] More severe blunt trauma may cause an aortic aneurysm or rupture of the aorta at the ligamentum arteriosum, which may lead to hemomediastinum or hemothorax; these complications must be diagnosed immediately with aortography and corrected surgically.[30] Pneumothorax and hemothorax are often seen after chest trauma; signs of these complications should be assessed on the initial chest x-ray, and a thoracostomy tube should be placed as necessary.

Circulation

The final step of the initial resuscitation is to assess and support the circulation and blood pressure. It is crucial that systemic hypotension be prevented or rapidly corrected. Within the first few minutes, adequate IV access must be established,[15] usually by placing one or more peripheral IV catheters 18-gauge or larger. If the patient is severely hypotensive or in cardiac arrest, a cutdown over one or both ankles should be performed to cannulate the greater saphenous veins with 14- or 16-gauge catheters. Alternatively, a central venous pressure catheter may be inserted via the jugular or brachial veins to administer fluids and monitor central venous pressure.[30]

When IV access has been established, intravascular volume resuscitation should proceed as necessary to maintain or stabilize the blood pressure. If the blood pressure is stable from the outset, fluid resuscitation should be judicious to prevent overhydration, which may augment cerebral edema[30] and possibly lead to pulmonary edema, especially if there is an associated pulmonary contusion. Shock, if present, must be reversed as quickly and effectively as possible by restoring intravascular volume.[15]

In the trauma patient, hemorrhagic or hypovolemic (hematogenic) shock is most common.[5,30] Multiply injured patients may have additional causes of shock, such as a low cardiac output due to cardiac contusion or cardiac tamponade or a loss of peripheral vascular tone due to an injury of the cervical spinal cord. It is important to consider cardiogenic and neurogenic sources of shock, especially when the blood pressure does not respond to initial volume resuscitation. Absolute blood pressure may be a less accurate measure of shock than pulse rate, skin perfusion, and urine output because compensatory mechanisms may allow blood pressure to remain relatively stable during hemorrhage until profound volume loss causes it to fall abruptly.[15]

At San Francisco General Hospital, balanced salt (crystalloid) solutions, such as lactated Ringer's solution, are used for initial volume resuscitation.[7] Replacement of depleted extracellular fluid with lactated Ringer's solution has a significant benefit in the cellular and clinical response to shock.[7,28] Although colloidal solutions have long been used to treat shock or increased ICP, crystalloid solutions appear to have similar hemodynamic and pulmonary effects if given to the same hemodynamic end point.[15] Crystalloid solutions, however, tend to equilibrate rapidly with the interstitial space and therefore a greater volume will be required.

Experimental data suggest that increased serum glucose and IV glucose infusion may harm injured ischemic brain.[22,23] Therefore, unless serum hypoglycemia is present, crystalloid solutions with added glucose and particularly 50% dextrose solutions should be avoided in head-injured patients. If massive blood loss is evident, if serial measurements show a rapidly decreasing hematocrit, or if the blood pressure remains low after infusion of 2 L of crystalloid solution,[30] type-specific or, preferably, cross-matched blood should be transfused. The hematocrit should be approximately 32%–35% to ensure optimal perfusion and oxygen carrying capacity.[15] All solutions and blood should be warmed before infusion to avoid causing cardiac arrhythmias from rapid infusion of cold fluids.[30]

As hemorrhagic shock is being treated with volume expansion, the hemorrhage must quickly be found and controlled.[15] Common sites of bleeding include the chest, abdomen, pelvis, and areas adjacent to fractures of long bones, such as the femur. Hemothorax and hemoperitoneum may require urgent surgical intervention in the operating room; bleeding adjacent to fractures is usually self-limited but may cause a compartment syndrome, necessitating intervention. These problems should be treated by the appropriate specialist while the neurosurgeon attends to the severe head injury and transtentorial herniation.

Other Measures

Mannitol

We routinely administer mannitol, 1–1.5 g/kg IV, as soon as possible after admission, to all severely head-injured patients as an additional means of lowering suspected elevations in ICP (Table 4-2). Mannitol is administered whether or not there are clinical signs of transtentorial herniation. A 6-carbon sugar similar to glucose, mannitol is not metabolized; and because it does not cross the normal blood-brain barrier, it remains predominantly in the intravascular and extracerebral extracellular space.[11] Wise and Chater[35] were

Table 4-2 Initial Management of Severe Head Injury

Obtain lateral cervical and anteroposterior chest radiographs
Place Foley catheter
If blood pressure is stable, administer mannitol, 1–1.5 g/kg IV
Keep cervical spine immobilized until radiographs have been reviewed and cervical spinal injuries have been ruled out

the first to show that mannitol given by rapid IV infusion decreases cerebrospinal fluid pressure and brain mass. The traditional view held that infusion of hypertonic mannitol into the intravascular space resulted in osmotic dehydration of the brain and reduced the volume of extracellular free water.[26] However, mannitol also improves intracranial compliance out of proportion to its effect on ICP.[14]

Mannitol infusion has several additional effects: it results in immediate volume expansion, which increases systemic arterial blood pressure,[35] and hemodilution, which reduces blood viscosity.[6,19] It also increases the deformability of red blood cells, which improves blood viscosity unrelated to hemodilution.[6] Muizelaar et al.[19] showed experimentally that cerebral vasoconstriction occurs in response to the mannitol-induced decrease in blood viscosity. They proposed that decreased blood viscosity leads to improved red cell oxygen transport and, when CO_2 responsiveness is intact, results in vasoconstriction.[18,19] Rosner and Coley[26] have shown that ICP responds better to mannitol in patients with a low initial cerebral perfusion pressure than in those with an initially high perfusion pressure. They postulate that the effect of mannitol on systemic arterial blood pressure increases cerebral perfusion pressure and allows direct cerebral vasoconstriction. Thus, mannitol infusion may result in cerebral vasoconstriction and decrease ICP through several mechanisms independent of its osmotic effect. If the patient is initially hypotensive (systolic blood pressure less than 80 mm Hg), mannitol infusion should be delayed until the blood pressure has been restored.

Furosemide

Furosemide has long been used to reduce intracerebral free water and brain edema.[8,27] It appears to act, in part, by establishing an intravascular diuresis, which increases intravascular oncotic pressure and thus extracts extracellular free water from the brain.[27] It may also reduce the production of cerebrospinal fluid.[25] Furosemide in combination with mannitol reportedly reduces ICP more effectively than either drug alone.[8,25,27,34] Roberts et al.[25] showed experimentally that administration of furosemide 15 minutes after infusion of mannitol resulted in the most profound and sustained reduction of elevated ICP. This synergistic effect did not appear to result from an alteration in the renal excretion of mannitol. Alternatively, furosemide may help sustain either the elevated serum osmolality or the osmotic gradient across the blood-brain barrier induced by mannitol.[31]

At present, furosemide is considered by some authors to be potentially useful in the treatment of elevated ICP after head injury.[17] In combination, furosemide and mannitol may cause rapid dehydration, which is likely to be detrimental to patients with multiple injuries. Patients with unstable vital signs or systemic hypotension (systolic blood pressure below 80 mm Hg) should generally not be treated with diuretics, which could cause further instability of the blood pressure from dehydration and further decrease cerebral perfusion pressure.

Summary

The goals of initial management of the patient with traumatic transtentorial herniation are the same as those for all severely head-injured patients. First, an airway must be established without exacerbating possible cervical spinal injuries. The patient may then be hyperventilated to correct hypoxia, lower $PaCO_2$, and decrease ICP. The circulation must be assessed; if present, shock should be treated with rapid volume resuscitation using crystalloid solutions. The cause of shock should be determined and treated; this may require thoracotomy or laparotomy. Chest and abdominal injuries must be identified and treated. Finally, mannitol should be administered by IV infusion. Hyperventilation and mannitol may decrease elevated ICP and therefore improve cerebral perfusion pressure, potentially allowing the brain to better accommodate an intracranial mass lesion until it can be identified and treated directly.

References

1. Andrews BT, Pitts LH, Lovely MP, et al.: Is computed tomographic scanning necessary in patients with tentorial herniation? Results of immediate surgical exploration without com-

puted tomography in 100 patients. Neurosurgery 19:408-413, 1986.

2. Aprahamian C, Thompson DM, Finger WA: Experimental cervical spine injury model: evaluation of airway management and splinting techniques. Ann Emerg Med 13:21-24, 1984.
3. Baker CC, Thomas AN, Trunkey DD: The role of emergency room thoracotomy in trauma. J Trauma 20:848-855, 1980.
4. Bivins HG, Ford S, Bezmalinovic Z, et al.: The effect of axial traction during orotracheal intubation of the trauma victim with an unstable cervical spine. Ann Emerg Med 17:25-29, 1988.
5. Blalock A: Shock: further studies with particular reference to effects of hemorrhage. Arch Surg 29:837-857 1934.
6. Burke AM, Quest DO, Chien S, et al.: The effects of mannitol on blood viscosity. J Neurosurg 55:550-553, 1981.
7. Canizaro PC, Prager MD, Shires GT: The infusion of Ringer's lactate solution during shock. Changes in lactate, excess lactate, and pH. Am J Surg 122:650-644, 1971.
8. Cottrell JE, Robustelli A, Post K: Furosemide- and mannitol-induced changes in intracranial pressure and serum osmolality and electrolytes. Anesthesiology 47:28-30, 1977.
9. Doolan LA, O'Brien JF: Safe intubation in cervical spine injury. Anaesth Intensive Care 13:319-324, 1985.
10. Fletcher SA, Henderson LT, Miner ME, et al.: The successful surgical removal of intracranial nasogastric tubes. J Trauma 27: 948-952, 1987.
11. Langfitt TW: Increased intracranial pressure and the cerebral circulation. In Youmans JR (ed): Neurological Surgery. Philadelphia: WB Saunders Co., 1982, pp 846-930.
12. Lassen NA: Brain extracellular pH: the main factor controlling cerebral blood flow. Scand J Clin Lab Invest 22:247-251, 1968.
13. Lassen NA: The luxury-perfusion syndrome and its possible relation to acute metabolic acidosis localized within the brain. Lancet 2:1113-1115, 1966.
14. Leech PJ, Miller JD: Intracranial volume-pressure relationships during experimental brain compression in primates. Part 3: the effect of mannitol and hypocapnia. J Neurol Neurosurg Psychiatry 37:1105-1111, 1974.
15. Lewis FR: Initial assessment and resuscitation: Symposium on Multiple Trauma. Emerg Med Clin North Am 2:733-748, 1984.
16. Lundberg N, Kjallquist A, Bien C: Reduction of increased intra-

cranial pressure by hyperventilation. Acta Psychiatr Scand (Suppl 34) 139:1-64, 1959.
17. Marshall LF, Marshall SB: Medical management of intracranial pressure. In Cooper PR (ed): Head Injury. 2nd ed. Baltimore, MD: Williams and Wilkins, 1987, pp 177-196.
18. Muizelaar JP, Lutz HA, Becker DP: Effect of mannitol on ICP and CBF and correlation with pressure autoregulation in severely head-injured patients. J Neurosurg 61:700-706, 1984.
19. Muizelaar JP, Wei EP, Kontos HA, et al.: Mannitol causes compensatory cerebral vasoconstriction and vasodilatation in response to blood viscosity changes. J Neurosurg 59:822-828, 1983.
20. O'Malley KF, Ross SE: The incidence of injury to the cervical spine in patients with craniocerebral injury. J Trauma 28:1476-1478, 1988.
21. Paul RL, Polanco O, Turney SZ, et al.: Intracranial pressure responses to alterations in arterial carbon dioxide pressure in patients with head injuries. J Neurosurg 36:714-720, 1972.
22. Rehncrona S, Rosen I, Siesjö B: Excessive cellular acidosis: an important mechanism of neuronal damage in the brain. Acta Physiol Scand 110:435-437, 1980.
23. Rehncrona S, Rosen I, Siesjö B: Brain lactic acidosis and ischemic cell damage: 1: Biochemistry and neurophysiology. J Cereb Blood Flow Metab 1:297-311, 1981.
24. Reivich M: Arterial P_{CO_2} and cerebral hemodynamics. Am J Physiol 206:25-35, 1964.
25. Roberts PA, Pollay M, Engles C, et al.: Effect on intracranial pressure of furosemide combined with varying doses and administration of mannitol. J Neurosurg 66:440-446, 1987.
26. Rosner MJ, Coley I: Cerebral perfusion pressure: a hemodynamic mechanism of mannitol and the postmannitol hemogram. Neurosurgery 21:147-156, 1987.
27. Schettini A, Stahurski B, Young HF: Osmotic and osmotic-loop diuresis in brain surgery. Effects on plasma and CSF electrolytes and ion secretion. J Neurosurg 56:679-684, 1982.
28. Shires GT, Coln D, Carrico J, et al.: Fluid therapy in hemorrhagic shock. Arch Surg 88:688-693, 1964.
29. Smith JP, Bodai BI, Aubourg R, et al.: A field evaluation of the esophageal obturator airway. J Trauma 23:317-321, 1983.
30. Thal ER: Initial management of the multiply injured patient. In

Cooper PR (ed): Head Injury. 2nd ed. Baltimore, MD: Williams and Wilkins, 1987, pp 34-50.

31. Tsutsumi H, Ide K, Mizutani T, et al.: The relationship between intracranial pressure, cerebral perfusion pressure and outcome in head-injured patient: the critical level of cerebral perfusion pressure. In Miller JD, Teasdale GM, Rowan JO, et al. (eds): ICP VI. Berlin: Springer-Verlag, 1985, pp 661-666.
32. Wang JF, Reves JG, Gutierrez FA: Awake fiberoptic laryngoscopic tracheal intubation for anterior cervical cord trauma. Int Surg 64:69-72, 1979.
33. Weiss MH: Mid- and lower cervical spine injuries. In Wilkins RH, Rengachary SS (eds): Neurosurgery. New York: McGraw-Hill, 1986, pp 1708-1715.
34. Wilkinson HA, Wepsic JG, Austin G: Diuretic synergy in the treatment of acute experimental cerebral edema. J Neurosurg 34:203-208, 1971.
35. Wise BL, Chater N: The value of hypertonic mannitol solution in decreasing brain mass and lowering cerebrospinal fluid pressure. J Neurosurg 19:1038-1043, 1962.

CHAPTER 5

The Effect of Systemic Hypotension and Hypoxia on the Neurological Examination

Systemic abnormalities such as hypotension or cardiac arrest and hypoxia are common after severe head injury. In the series of Miller et al.,[26] 13% of patients were hypotensive and 30% were hypoxic upon arrival in the emergency room. Andrews et al.[2] reported that 38% of patients with evident brain stem dysfunction after head injury had systemic hypotension or were in cardiac arrest at admission. In head-injured adults, systemic hypotension is often due to hemorrhagic hypotension as a consequence of blood loss from systemic injuries.[25] Other potential causes of systemic hypotension include dysfunction of cardiovascular reflex centers in the medulla,[7] spinal cord injury causing loss of sympathetic tone, or a myocardial insult, such as a cardiac contusion or myocardial infarction, at the time of head injury.[11]

Hypoxia and systemic hypotension decrease the survival rate and worsen the outcome after head injury.[8,25,26,34] When severe, these systemic abnormalities can cause central nervous system ischemia, which can alter or suppress brain stem reflexes and higher cortical function.[7,18,22,23] Because the neurological findings at admission are used to define the severity of head injury and to select subsequent diagnostic studies and treatment, it is critically important that the neurological examination accurately reflect intracranial

From *Traumatic Transtentorial Herniation and Its Management* by Brian T. Andrews, MD and Lawrence H. Pitts, MD © 1991, Futura Publishing Co., Inc., Mount Kisco, NY.

pathology. In patients with head injury, the degree of systemic hypotension or hypoxia that would depress neurological function as a result of ischemia has previously been unclear. Because of the loss of cerebrovascular autoregulation that accompanies head injury[6,24,30] and the adverse effect of intracranial mass lesions on local cerebral blood flow,[21] head-injured patients may be especially sensitive to systemic hypotension or hypoxia.

Cardiac Arrest and Systemic Hypotension

We recently evaluated the effect of systemic hypotension or cardiac arrest on the neurological examination in patients with severe head injury to determine if the clinical signs of mechanical brain compression remain valid indicators of brain compression due to transtentorial herniation.[1] We also sought to ascertain the level of systemic hypotension below which the neurological examination no longer reflects the presence of an intracranial mass lesion. The study was performed by correlating the initial neurological findings, the results of surgery and computerized tomography (CT), and the clinical course of 36 patients admitted with signs of upper brain stem dysfunction who had varying degrees of systemic hypotension or were resuscitated from cardiac arrest after severe head injury. The initial resuscitation and management have been described in detail.[1]

Each patient was taken directly to the operating room for emergency bilateral burr-hole exploration. Upon discovery of a significant intracranial hematoma, the exposure was converted into a large craniotomy, and the lesion was evacuated. All patients whose cardiovascular status was stable underwent CT scanning of the brain immediately after the operation. An autopsy was performed on all patients who died in the operating room or in the early postoperative period. The autopsy reports were reviewed for acute intracranial hematomas not found during burr-hole exploration.

At admission, 10 patients were being resuscitated from cardiac arrest, seven had a systolic blood pressure (SBP) less than 60 mm Hg, and 19 had an SBP of 60–90 mm Hg. The diastolic blood pressure was usually not recorded, and therefore mean blood pressure could not be determined. Eighteen patients (50%) had major chest, abdominal, or orthopedic injuries or underwent a thoracotomy in the emergency room.

Table 5-1 Neurological Findings at Admission According to Initial Systolic Blood Pressure

		Systolic Blood Pressure (mm Hg)	
Findings	*Cardiac Arrest (n = 10)*	*< 60 (n = 7)*	*60–90 (n = 19)*
Anisocoria	4	2	9
Bilaterally unreactive pupils	6	5	10
Absent corneal reflexes	10	7	11
Hemiparesis	0	0	4
Abnormal flexor/extensor posturing	1	0	4
Flaccid	9	7	11

The neurological findings are summarized in Table 5-1. The median Glasgow coma score was 3 (range 3–8). Four of the 10 patients in cardiac arrest had anisocoria (40%), and six had bilaterally unreactive pupils. All 10 patients had absent corneal reflexes; nine were flaccid and one had bilateral flexor posturing. Two (29%) of seven patients with an initial SBP less than 60 mm Hg had anisocoria and five had bilaterally unreactive pupils; all had absent corneal reflexes and all were flaccid. Nine (47%) of 19 patients with an initial SBP of 60 mm Hg or greater had anisocoria, and 10 had bilaterally dilated unreactive pupils; eight had active corneal reflexes, and four had a hemiparesis.

The surgical findings are shown in Table 5-2. Only one (10%) of 10 patients resuscitated from cardiac arrest had a significant extra-axial hematoma. This patient had anisocoria, and the hematoma was ipsilateral to the larger pupil. Only one (14%) of seven patients with an initial SBP of less than 60 mm Hg had a hematoma. This patient had bilaterally dilated and unreactive pupils, no corneal reflexes, and was flaccid. No patient with an SBP less than 60 mm Hg and lateralizing neurological findings had an intracranial mass lesion. In contrast, 13 (68%) of 19 patients with an initial SBP of 60 mm Hg or greater had extra-axial hematomas; and seven (78%) of nine patients with anisocoria had extra-axial hematomas, all of which were ipsilateral to the dilated pupil.

Thus, extra-axial hemorrhages were significantly more common among patients with an initial SBP of 60 mm Hg or greater than among those with a lower blood pressure or initial cardiac arrest

Table 5-2 Surgical Findings According to Initial Systolic Blood Pressure

Findings	Cardiac Arrest (n = 10)	Systolic Blood Pressure (mm Hg) < 60 (n = 7)	Systolic Blood Pressure (mm Hg) 60–90 (n = 19)
Significant hematoma	1 (10%)	1 (14%)	13 (68%)*
Hematoma ipsilateral to the larger pupil	1/4 (25%)	0	7/9 (78%)†

*$p < 0.01$; †$p < 0.05$.

($p < 0.01$). Anisocoria was also associated with an ipsilateral intracranial hematoma more frequently in patients with an initial SBP of at least 60 mm Hg than in those in the other two groups ($p < 0.05$). In all patients with an initial SBP of 60 mm Hg or greater who had positive burr-hole explorations, the hemorrhage was ipsilateral to the dilated pupil. The presence of hemiparesis did not help to determine the side of the hematoma.

Systemic hypotension worsens the prognosis for recovery after head injury.[4,8,26,28] The added morbidity may result from associated systemic injuries, injury to the brain from decreased cerebral perfusion,[28] or less often, direct injury to cardiovascular reflex centers in the medulla.[7] Hypotension may exacerbate cerebral ischemia resulting from increased intracranial pressure and mechanical compression caused by acute intracranial hematomas.[1,33]

Cerebral autoregulation normally maintains cerebral blood flow if arterial pressure remains greater than approximately 60 mm Hg. Below this level, blood flow to the brain decreases linearly with falling blood pressure, and cerebral ischemia occurs.[10,24] The loss of cerebral autoregulation that has been reported to occur with severe head injury[6,24,30] may result in decreased cerebral blood flow and ischemia at even lesser degrees of systemic hypotension. The results of the study reviewed above, however, indicate that the neurological findings in head-injured patients accurately reflect the presence of intracranial mass lesions despite SBP as low as 60 mm Hg. In such patients, cerebral autoregulation may not have been severely altered. When the initial SBP was less than 60 mm Hg or when the patient was admitted in cardiac arrest, however, the neurological examination probably did not reflect mechanical brain compression as much as generalized brain ischemia.

These findings have important implications for the treatment of severe head injury. In patients with SBP of 60 mm Hg or greater, anisocoria usually indicates mechanical brain compression. Diagnostic studies and treatment should be pursued without delay.[2] In patients who initially are in cardiac arrest or have SBP less than 60 mm Hg, the neurological examination does not reliably indicate mechanical brain compression from an intracranial mass lesion. Therefore, unless other systemic injuries necessitate immediate operative intervention, cranial CT scanning should be performed while resuscitation is continued, and further neurosurgical treatment should be predicated on the information obtained.

Systemic Hypoxia

Systemic hypoxia appears to be an even more common complication of severe head injury than systemic hypotension.[20,25,26,35] Katsurada et al.[20] reported that among patients in coma after head injury, 43% had arterial hypoxemia below 70 mm Hg, 51% had an alveolar-arterial oxygen difference greater than 30 mm Hg, 14% had hypercarbia above 45 mm Hg, and 20% had an arterial pH below 7.35. In the series of Miller et al.,[26] 30% of severely head-injured patients had an initial arterial oxygen tension (PaO_2) of 65 mm Hg or less. Similarly, Sinha et al.[35] reported that 20% of their patients with head and spinal cord injuries had an initial PaO_2 of 60 mm Hg or less. Systemic hypoxia may result from the immediate onset of apnea after head injury,[25] subsequent abnormal breathing patterns,[30] hypoventilation due to an associated spinal cord injury causing paralysis of thoracic musculature, airway obstruction due to facial or neck injuries, direct injury to the chest wall or lungs, or fat emboli in the pulmonary circulation.[33,35]

The effect of systemic hypoxia on the neurological examination has most often been evaluated clinically in the setting of acute airway obstruction, suffocation, and drowning. Systemic hypotension usually accompanies hypoxia owing to the latter's effect on the myocardium and vascular bed.[31] Thus, cerebral ischemia may result from both systemic hypoxia and hypoperfusion. However, if systemic hypotension is meticulously treated, humans can tolerate extremely low PaO_2 without obvious neurological manifestations and without sequelae. In the series of Gray and Horner,[9] eight of 22 patients with a PaO_2 of 20 mm Hg or less at admission were alert, seven were somnolent, and seven were comatose. Thirteen (59%) survived, 10 in good condition. One young man who was apneic and comatose, with a PaO_2 of 7 mm Hg, recovered and eventually had a good outcome. In that study, the level of consciousness did not correlate well with the PCO_2,[9] although others have noted that neurological function is poor and recovery unusual when arterial hypoxia of 20 mm Hg or less is associated with hypercarbia.[32]

Severe hypoxia may cause clinical signs of a metabolic encephalopathy, including progressive alterations in consciousness leading to coma,[31] changes in respiratory patterns,[29] and tremors, asterixis, myoclonus, and flexor or extensor posturing. Usually the brain stem reflexes remain intact until profound anoxia has occurred, at which time pupillary dilatation and loss of oculocephalic reflexes may occur.[31]

Experimentally, acute anoxia has been shown to produce pupillary constriction until the cardiac output has been reduced by 70%. The pupils then dilate and remain dilated until several minutes after death, when they return to the midposition.[5] Pupillary dilatation has also been documented after 2–6 minutes of asphyxia or after ventilation with gas mixtures containing only 5%–7% oxygen.[12] Pupillary dilatation during hypoxia despite sympathetic and parasympathetic denervation[19] suggests that a direct effect of hypoxia or other factors circulating in the bloodstream, as well as neural input, are involved in the dilatatory response. Nevertheless, during profound hypoxia, the pupils may remain small or in the midposition until the time of death.[17]

Ishige et al.[14] showed in rats that a hypoxic episode (PaO_2 of 35–40 mm Hg for 30 minutes) immediately after a fluid-percussion injury caused prolonged unresponsiveness initially and significantly worsened neurological function 24 hours later compared with impact injury alone. Additional studies of this model showed that rats subjected to hypoxia had increased cerebral edema,[13] worsened high-energy phosphate metabolism,[15] reduced cerebral blood flow,[13] and more extensive histopathological damage[14] compared with rats subjected to fluid-percussion injury alone. Nelson et al.[27] found that severe hypoxia delayed the neurological recovery and worsened the outcome of cats with similar head injuries. Jenkins et al.[16] demonstrated that even relatively mild degrees of experimental head injury cause more prolonged neurological deficits when hypoxia is also present. Thus, experimental findings show that hypoxia after severe head injury can significantly alter immediate neurological function, but its effects on brain stem function have not been documented in severely head-injured humans.

Summary

Although even severe degrees of systemic hypoxia may be tolerated with few neurological abnormalities in healthy humans, profound hypoxia causes profound alterations in consciousness and subsequently in brain stem function. Systemic hypoxia is a common complication of severe head injury, and experimental models indicate that hypoxia after severe head injury worsens the immediate and subsequent neurological examinations. The degree of this effect has not been documented in head-injured humans. Systemic hypotension during the hypoxic episode may further depress neurological function. It is likely that neurological abnormalities in the hypoxic (and hypotensive) severely head-injured patient may be significantly depressed by these metabolic insults. Therefore, the findings of the initial neurological examination in such cases should not be the sole basis for major treatment decisions, such as the placement of exploratory burr-holes. Additional diagnostic studies, such as CT brain scans should be performed, and further treatment guided by the findings.

References

1. Andrews BT, Levy ML, Pitts LH: Implications of systemic hypotension for the neurological examination in patients with severe head injury. Surg Neurol 28:419-422, 1987.
2. Andrews BT, Pitts LH, Lovely MP, et al.: Is computed tomographic scanning necessary in patients with tentorial herniation? Results of immediate surgical exploration in 100 patients. Neurosurgery 19:408-413, 1986.
3. Baker CC, Caronna JJ, Trunkey DD: Neurological outcome after emergency room thoracotomy. Am J Surg 139:677-681, 1980.
4. Becker DP, Miller JD, Sweet RC, et al.: Head injury management.

In Popp AJ, Bourke RS, Nelson LR (eds): Neural Trauma. New York: Raven Press, 1979, pp 313-328.

5. Binnion PF, McFarland RJ: The relationship of cardiac massage and pupil size in cardiac arrest in dogs. Cardiovasc Res 3:915-917, 1967.
6. Bruce DA, Langfitt TW, Miller JD: Regional cerebral blood flow, intracranial pressure, and brain metabolism in comatose patients. J Neurosurg 38:131-144, 1973.
7. Cooper PR: Resuscitation of the multiply injured patient. Clin Neurosurg 29:225-239, 1981.
8. Eisenberg HM: Outcome after head injury: general considerations and neurobehavioral recovery. In: Becker DP, Povlishock JT (eds): Central Nervous System Trauma Status Report. Washington DC: National Institute of Neurological and Communicative Diseases and Stroke, 1985, pp 271-280.
9. Gray FD, Horner GJ: Survival following extreme hypoxemia. JAMA 211:1815-1817, 1970.
10. Harper AM: Autoregulation of cerebral blood flow: influence of arterial blood pressure on the flow through the cerebral cortex. J Neurol Neurosurg Psychiatry 29:398-403, 1966.
11. Hersch C: Electrocardiographic changes in head injuries. Circulation 23:853-860, 1961.
12. Hodes R: Efferent pathway for reflex pupillo-motor activity. Am J Physiol 131:144, 1940.
13. Ishige N, Pitts LH, Berry I, et al.: The effect of hypoxia on traumatic brain injury in rats: alterations in neurological function, brain edema, and cerebral blood flow. J Cereb Blood Flow Metab 7:759-767, 1987.
14. Ishige N, Pitts LH, Hashimoto T, et al.: Effect of hypoxia on traumatic brain injury in rats: Part 1. Changes in neurological function, electroencephalograms and histopathology. Neurosurgery 20:848-853, 1987.
15. Ishige N, Pitts LH, Pogliani L, et al.: Effect of hypoxia on traumatic brain injury in rats: Part 2. Changes in high-energy phosphate metabolism. Neurosurgery 20:854-858, 1987.
16. Jenkins LW, Lyeth BG, Hayes RL: The role of agonist-receptor interactions in the pathophysiology of mild and moderate head injury. In Fitch W, Barker J (eds): Mild to Moderate Head Injury. Amsterdam: Elsevier, 1985, pp 47-61.

17. Jordanov J, Ruben H: Reliability of pupillary changes as a clinical sign of hypoxia. Lancet 2:915-917, 1967.
18. Jorgensen EO, Malshow-Moller A: Cerebral prognostic signs during cardiopulmonary resuscitation. Resuscitation 6:217-225, 1978.
19. Kapp J, Paulson G: Pupillary changes induced by circulatory arrest. Neurology 16:225-229, 1966.
20. Katsurada K, Yamada R, Sugimoto T: Respiratory insufficiency in patients with severe head injury. Surgery 73:191-199, 1973.
21. Kingman TA, Mendelow AD, Graham DI, et al.: Experimental intracerebral mass: time-related effects on local cerebral blood flow. J Neurosurg 67:732-738, 1987.
22. Levy DE, Bates D, Caronna JJ, et al.: Prognosis in non-traumatic coma. Ann Intern Med 94:293-301, 1981.
23. Levy DE, Caronna JJ, Singer BH, et al.: Predicting outcome from hypoxic-ischemic coma. JAMA 253:1420-1426, 1985.
24. Lewelt W, Jenkins LW, Miller JD: Autoregulation of cerebral blood flow after experimental fluid-percussion injury of the brain. J Neurosurg 53:500-511, 1980.
25. Miller JD: Head injury and brain ischaemia-implications for therapy. Br J Anaesth 547:120-129, 1985.
26. Miller JD, Sweet RC, Narayan R, et al.: Early insults to the injured brain. JAMA 240:439-442, 1978.
27. Nelson LR, Auen EL, Bourke RS, et al.: A comparison of animal head injury models developed for treatment modality evaluation. In Grossman RG, Gildenberg PL (eds): Head Injury: Basic and Clinical Aspects. New York: Raven Press, 1982, pp 117-128.
28. Newfield P, Pitts LH, Kaktis J, et al.: The influence of shock on mortality after head injury. Crit Care Med 8:254-255, 1980.
29. North JB, Jennett S: Abnormal breathing patterns associated with acute brain damage. Arch Neurol 31:338-344, 1974.
30. Obrist WD, Langfitt TW, Jaggi JL, et al.: Cerebral blood flow and metabolism in comatose patients with acute head injury. J Neurosurg 61:241-253, 1984.
31. Plum F, Posner JB: The Diagnosis of Stupor and Coma. 3rd ed. Philadelphia, PA: FA Davis Co., 1980, pp 177-302.
32. Refsum HE: Relationship between state of consciousness and arterial hypoxemia and hypercapnia in patients with pulmonary insufficiency, breathing air. Clin Sci 25:361-367, 1963.

33. Riska EB, Myllynen P: Fat embolism in patients with multiple injuries. J Trauma 22:891-894, 1982.
34. Shimazu S, Shatney CH: Outcomes of trauma patients with no vital signs on hospital admission. J Trauma 23:312-316, 1983.
35. Sunha RP, Ducker TB, Perot PL: Arterial oxygenation. Findings and its significance in central nervous system trauma patients. JAMA 224:1258-1260, 1973.

CHAPTER 6

Neuroradiologic Evaluation

After the initial evaluation has been completed and the patient has been intubated, hyperventilated, and given intravenous mannitol, additional diagnostic studies to identify intracranial mass lesions must be selected. This decision is particularly important in patients with signs of transtentorial herniation, which usually results from brain stem compression caused by treatable extra-axial mass lesions.[4,10–13,16,20]

If the patient is hemodynamically unstable, has major penetrating thoracic or abdominal injuries, or appears to have significant ongoing blood loss, an exploratory laparotomy and, if necessary, a thoracotomy are almost invariably performed to control the bleeding.[14,23] In this setting it is impractical and unsafe to obtain additional diagnostic studies of the brain outside the operating room. During general surgical procedures, however, exploratory burr-holes may be placed in the frontal, temporal, and parietal regions bilaterally (see Chapter 7)[4] to identify extra-axial mass lesions; intraoperative ultrasonography may be performed to identify intraparenchymal lesions (see Chapter 9).[1] If a significant hematoma is discovered, it can be evacuated without delay.

If the patient is hemodynamically stable and does not have systemic injuries requiring urgent surgery, most head-injury experts recommend immediate computerized tomography (CT) of the brain.[7,8] Because of its relative speed, safety, and accuracy in identifying acute intra- and extra-axial hematomas, contusions, and brain swelling,[7,8,14] CT is the most important diagnostic modality for early assessment of the injured brain. Magnetic resonance imaging is not

From *Traumatic Transtentorial Herniation and Its Management* by Brian T. Andrews, MD and Lawrence H. Pitts, MD © 1991, Futura Publishing Co., Inc., Mount Kisco, NY.

useful for such assessment because of its relative unavailability, the time needed to perform a technically adequate study, and the poor resolution of acute hemorrhage and bone injury.[21]

Identification of an intracranial hemorrhage by CT depends upon the size and location of the lesion, whether the blood is mixed with cerebrospinal fluid (CSF) or brain parenchyma,[14] and when the scans are obtained relative to the time of trauma.[6] The radiographic density of blood is thought to reflect its hemoglobin content[17] and is highest immediately after hemorrhage. On CT scans, an acute hematoma appears as a brightly contrasting mass (60–90 Hounsfield units) compared with adjacent brain parenchyma and CSF (Fig. 6-1). The density gradually decreases as the blood clot is resorbed, becoming isointense with brain within a few days to weeks. A more chronic hemorrhage is hypointense compared with brain parenchyma.[6]

In patients with clinical signs of transtentorial herniation, CT scans may confirm the presence of brain stem compression by showing evidence of medial displacement of the temporal lobe, ranging from simple obliteration of the ambient cisterns (Fig. 6-2) to herniation of the uncus across the incisura.[9,18,19,22] The midbrain may appear to be shifted, rotated, or compressed (Figs. 6-3 and 6-4), and the aqueduct of Sylvius may be obliterated, causing early obstructive hydrocephalus. With more severe midline shift and compression of the ipsilateral and third ventricles, contralateral hydrocephalus may be seen (Fig. 6-4).[9,19] Central descending herniation of the brain stem may depress the pineal body,[9,19,22] but this finding is not well-demonstrated by CT. CT may also clarify unusual physical findings, such as a hemiparesis ipsilateral to the dilated pupil, which usually indicates a Kernohan's notch phenomenon (Fig. 6-5).[18]

When the initial CT findings suggest transtentorial herniation after head injury, the clinical outcome is worse than when such findings are absent. Toutant et al.[24] found that obliteration of the basal cisterns was associated with a poorer outcome than when they remained open. In their series of 218 severely head-injured patients, the mortality rates were 77%, 39%, and 22% in those with CT scans showing absent, compressed, and normal cisterns, respectively. This association was statistically even more significant after adjustment for the initial Glasgow coma score. Among patients with a relatively high score of 6 to 8, nearly 80% of those with absent cisterns had a poor outcome (severely disabled, vegetative, or dead) compared with

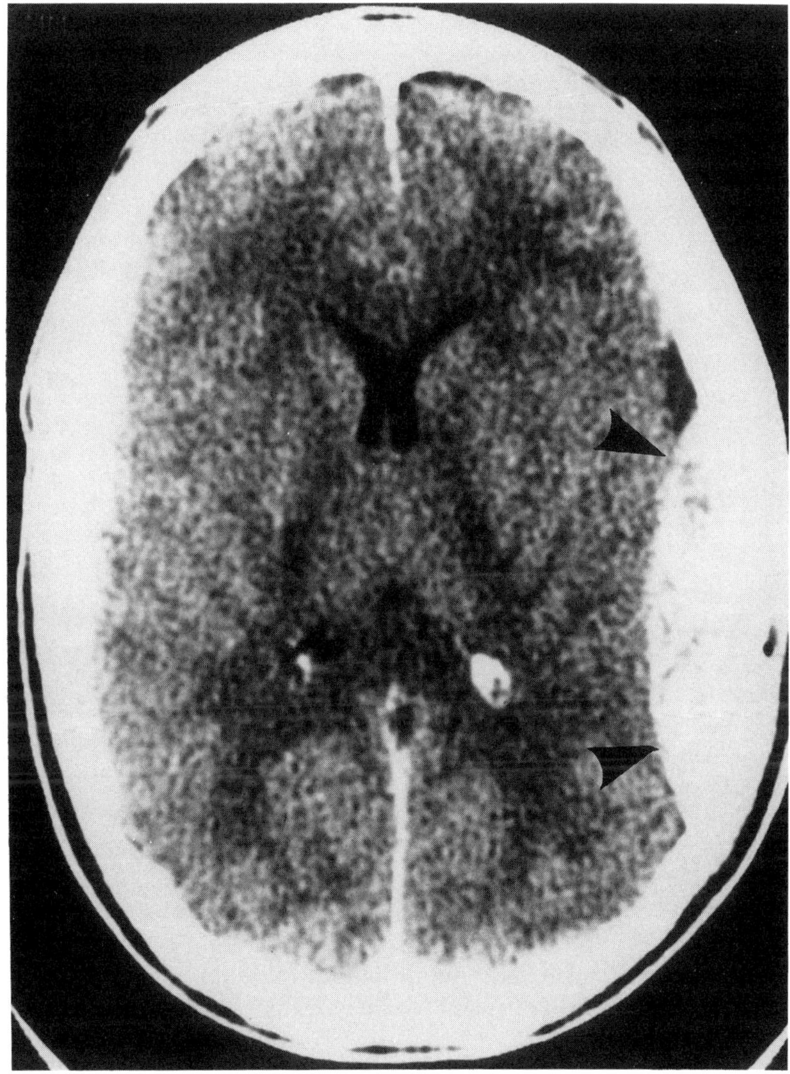

Figure 6-1. CT scan showing an acute epidural hemorrhage as an area of bright contrast *(arrowheads)* compared with brain parenchyma.

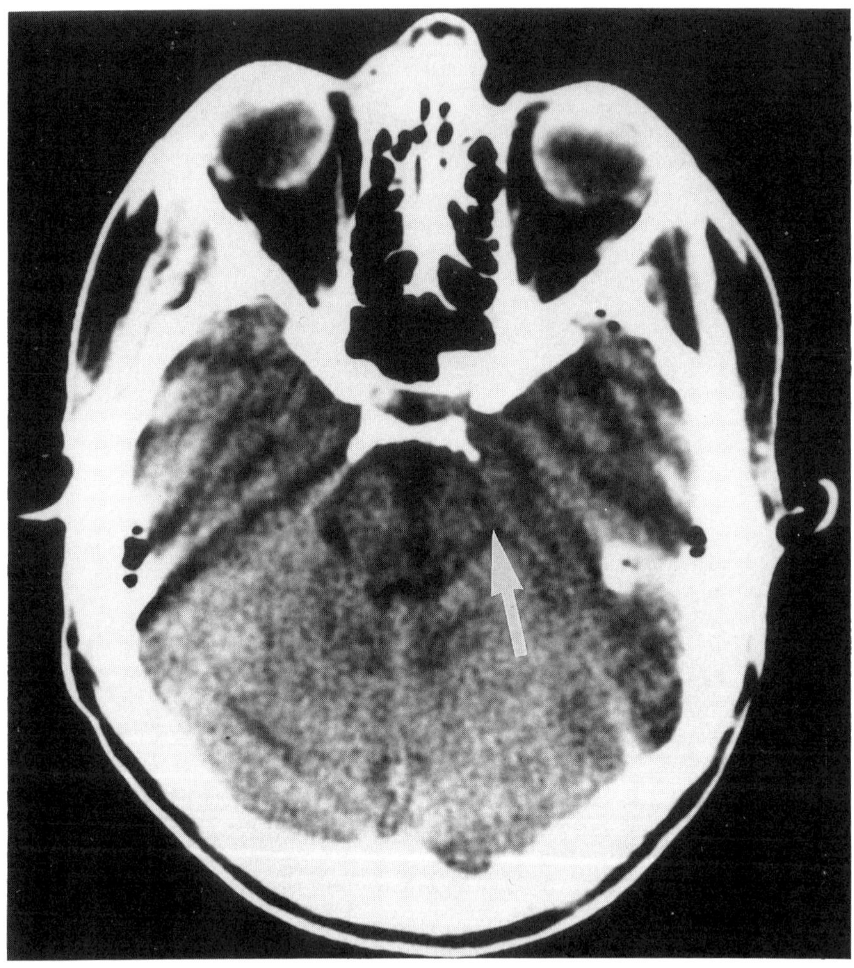

Figure 6-2. CT scan showing unilateral obliteration of the ambient cistern *(arrow)* caused by early transtentorial herniation of the uncus.

only 20% of those with normal cisterns ($p < 0.001$). All patients in whom CT scans showed absent cisterns and a midline shift greater than 15 mm died. Although absence of the basal cisterns was associated with severely increased intracranial pressure, direct brain

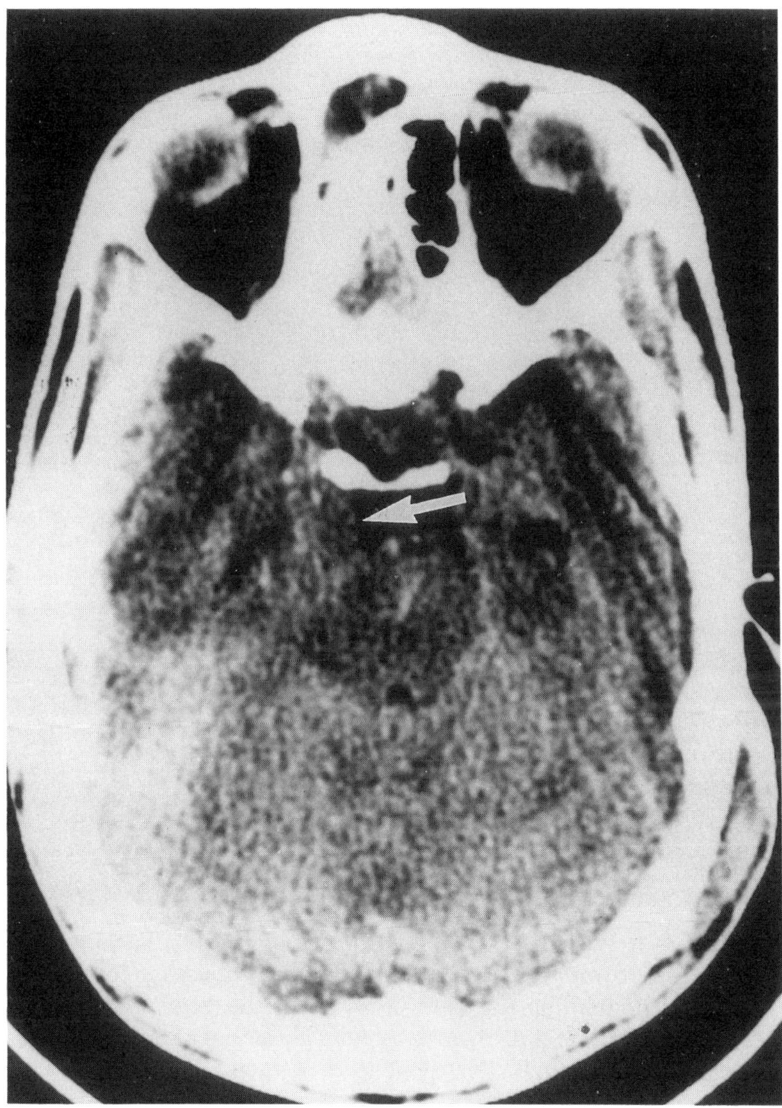

Figure 6-3. CT scan showing severe unilateral transtentorial herniation of the uncus *(arrow)* and brain stem compression.

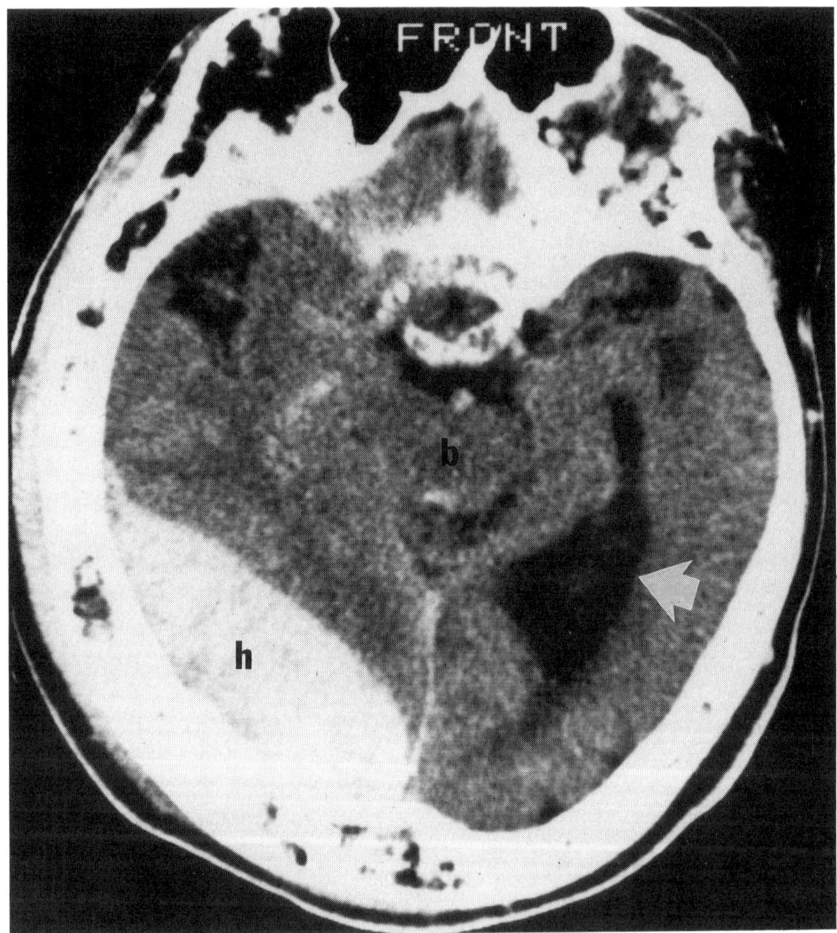

Figure 6-4. CT scan showing transtentorial herniation with compression and rotation of the brain stem (b) caused by a large occipital hematoma (h). Compression of the ventricle ipsilateral to the mass and destruction of the aqueduct of Sylvius have resulted in contralateral hydrocephalus *(arrow)*.

stem compression was probably an additional reason for the higher morbidity and mortality rates.

The initial CT findings may also predict which patients are at greater risk for developing clinical brain stem compression after se-

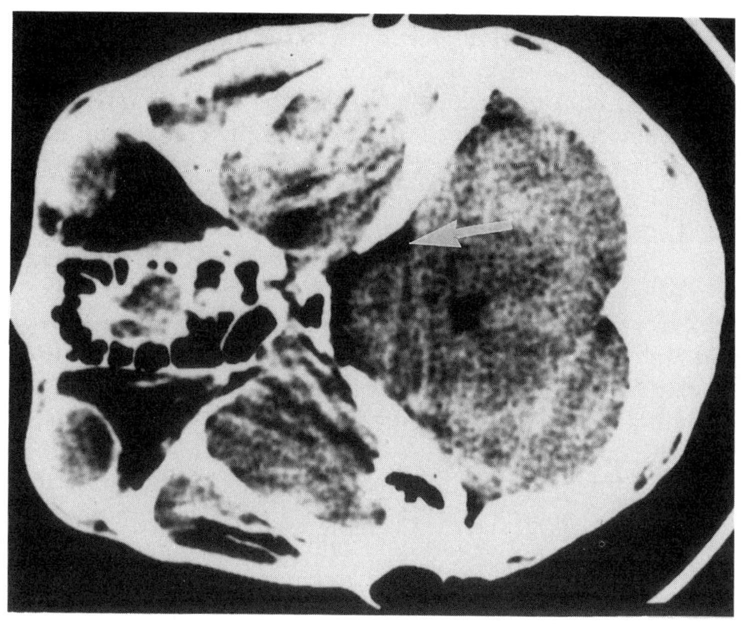

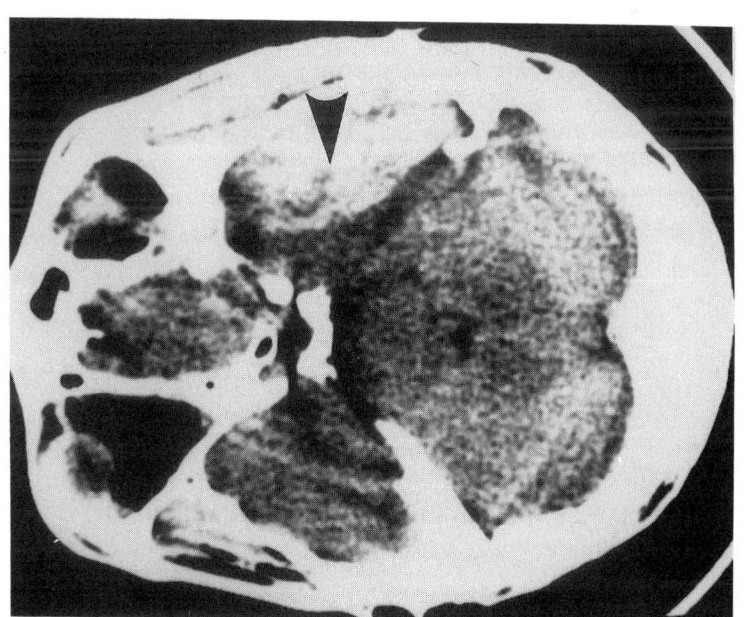

Figure 6-5. CT brain scans obtained at two different levels in a patient with Kernohan's notch phenomenon. The brain stem has been displaced along with the cerebral hemispheres away from the side of a mass lesion *(arrowhead)*, widening the ipsilateral ambient cistern *(arrow)* and compressing the contralateral cerebral peduncle against the edge of the tentorium.

vere head injury. Intracerebral hemorrhages in the temporal lobe are much more likely to cause clinical signs of transtentorial herniation than those in the frontal or parieto-occipital lobe[2] (see Chapter 8). Temporal lobe hematomas may lead to signs of brain stem compression even in the absence of elevated intracranial pressure.[15]

Although CT scans provide valuable diagnostic and prognostic information, there are several disadvantages to obtaining them immediately after the initial evaluation and resuscitation. Even when a scanner and a technician are readily available, it usually takes 25–40 minutes to complete the scan. In many hospitals, where a technician is not immediately available, the delay may be much longer. During this critical period, the only options for treating potential ongoing brain stem compression are to continue hyperventilation and mannitol administration. Moreover, while the patient is isolated within the scanner, it is difficult to monitor blood pressure closely, observe the airway, or reassess neurological status. If a significant complication such as systemic hypotension develops, it may remain undetected and untreated until the scan has been completed. Such complications can have profound implications, especially among patients with brain stem compression due to transtentorial herniation. Finally, CT scans obtained soon after admission may not show an obvious mass. In a small percentage of patients, a significant intracranial hematoma may develop minutes or hours later.[4] In such cases, an initially negative scan may lull the unwary clinician into a false sense of security.

We emphatically support the use of CT to evaluate all severely head-injured patients *without* signs of transtentorial herniation. CT is also indispensable for reevaluating patients who have delayed deterioration after head injury. However, we question the practice of *invariably* obtaining CT scans at the first opportunity in patients with signs of brain stem compression at admission or during the initial evaluation.[4] Such patients have a high incidence of significant intracranial mass lesions, most of which are in the epi- or subdural space.[3-5,10-13,16,20] This fact remains true regardless of age or injury mechanism[3–5] except among patients with severe systemic hypotension (initial systolic blood pressure less than 60 mm Hg) or cardiac arrest[3] and among young adults injured in high-speed motor-vehicle accidents.[4]

It is our policy, therefore, that most patients with obvious signs of transtentorial herniation after head injury undergo CT scanning after complete bilateral burr-hole exploration, as described in the next chapter. It should be emphasized, however, that many neurotrauma experts recommend obtaining a CT scan as soon as possible in *all* patients with severe head injury, whether or not signs of brain stem compression are present, and predicating further management upon the results obtained.

References

1. Andrews BT, Bederson J, Pitts LH: Use of intraoperative ultrasonography to improve the diagnostic accuracy of exploratory burr-holes in patients with traumatic tentorial herniation. Neurosurgery 24:345-347, 1989.
2. Andrews BT, Chiles B, Pitts LH: The effect of intracerebral hematoma location on the risk of tentorial herniation and clinical outcome. J Neurosurg 69:518-522, 1988.
3. Andrews BT, Levy M, Pitts LH: Implications of systemic hypotension for the initial neurological examination in patients with severe head injury. Surg Neurol 28:419-422, 1987.
4. Andrews BT, Pitts LH, Lovely MP, et al.: Is CT scanning necessary in patients with tentorial herniation? Results of immediate surgical exploration without computerized tomography in 100 patients. Neurosurgery 19:408-414, 1986.
5. Andrews BT, Ross AM, Pitts LH: Surgical exploration before computed tomographic scanning in children with traumatic tentorial herniation. Surg Neurol 32:434-438, 1989.
6. Bergstrom M, Ericson K, Levander B, et al.: Computed tomography of cranial subdural and epidural hematomas: variations of attenuation related to time and clinical events such as rebleeding. J Comput Assist Tomogr 1:449-455, 1977.
7. Bruce DA, Gennarelli A, Langfitt W: Resuscitation from coma due to head injury. Crit Care Med 6:254-269, 1978.
8. Clifton GL: Early management in the emergency room and operating room. Neurol Clin 4:18-24, 1982.
9. Hahn F, Gurney J: CT signs of central descending transtentorial herniation. Am J NR 6:844-845, 1985.
10. Howell DA: Upper brain stem compression and foraminal impaction with intracranial space-occupying lesions and brain swelling. Brain 82:525-550, 1959.

11. Jefferson G: Tentorial pressure cone. Arch Neurol Psychiatry 40:857-876, 1940.
12. Jennett WB, Stern WE: Tentorial herniation, the midbrain and the pupil. Experimental studies in brain compression. J Neurosurg 17:598-609, 1960.
13. Johnson RT, Yates PO: Clinico-pathological aspects of pressure changes at the tentorium. Acta Radiol 46:242-249, 1956.
14. Kishore PRS, Hall JA: Radiographic evaluation. In Cooper PR (ed): Head Injury. 2nd ed. Baltimore, MD: Williams and Wilkins, 1987, pp 51-71.
15. Marshall LF, Cotten JM, Bowers-Marshall S, et al.: Pupillary abnormalities, elevated intracranial pressure and mass lesion location. In Miller JD, Teasdale GM, Rowan JO, et al. (eds): Intracranial Pressure VI. Berlin: Springer-Verlag, 1986.
16. Meyer A: Herniation of the brain. Arch Neurol Psychiatry 4: 387-400, 1920.
17. New PF, Aronow S: Attenuation measurements of whole blood and blood fractions in computerized tomography. Radiology 121:635-640, 1970.
18. Pitts LH: Neurological evaluation of the head injury patient. Clin Neurosurg 29:203-224, 1981.
19. Ropper AH: Lateral displacement of the brain and level of consciousness in patients with an acute hemispheral mass. N Engl J Med 314:953-958, 1986.
20. Schwartz GA, Rosner AA: Displacement and herniation of hippocampal gyrus through the incisura tentorii: a clinicopathological study. Arch Neurol Psychiatry 46:297-321, 1941.
21. Snow RB, Zimmerman RD, Gandy SE, et al.: Comparison of magnetic resonance imaging and computed tomography in the evaluation of head injury. Neurosurgery 18:45-52, 1986.
22. Stovring J: Descending transtentorial herniation: findings on computed tomography. Neuroradiology 14:101-104, 1977.
23. Thal ER, McClelland RN, Shires GT: Abdominal trauma. In Shires GT (ed): Care of the Trauma Patient. 2nd ed. New York: McGraw-Hill Book Co., 1979, pp 290-348.
24. Toutant SM, Klauber MR, Marshall LF, et al.: Absent or compressed basal cisterns on first CT scan: ominous predictors of outcome in severe head injury. J Neurosurg 61:691-694, 1984.

CHAPTER 7

Emergency Burr-Hole Exploration

Clinical signs of brain stem compression after severe head injury indicate an expanding intracranial hematoma in up to 70% of cases.[3,4,6,9-11,17,27] Without treatment, compression from a mass lesion will probably cause irreversible brain stem injury. Most acute traumatic intracranial hematomas are extra-axial and therefore likely to be discovered by properly performed burr-hole exploration. In several large series of patients with severe head injury, subdural hematomas constituted 42%–71% and epidural hematomas 7%–34% of acute mass lesions.[3–5,7,9,10,13,15] Intracerebral hematomas, which may be missed by immediate burr-hole exploration, are rare immediately after injury; they generally develop in the subsequent hours or days.[1,3,20] Interhemispheric subdural hematomas are also rare.[19]

Prompt diagnosis and evacuation of the hematoma can minimize injury from displacement of the brain and from increased intracranial pressure (ICP).[3] Although the overall prognosis after transtentorial herniation is poor,[3,9–11,22,25,26] a good outcome is possible in many cases.[3,6,8–10,23,24,26,27] Seeking to speed the diagnosis and treatment of intracranial hematomas without interrupting direct intensive monitoring or management of life-threatening systemic injury, we have for many years performed diagnostic burr-hole exploration before obtaining computerized tomography (CT) scans in all patients admitted to the emergency room with clinical signs of transtentorial herniation or brain stem compression after severe head injury.[10,17,21,29] In 1986, we reported the results of burr-hole exploration in 100 consecutive patients with traumatic transtentorial herniation.[3] Since then, 53

From *Traumatic Transtentorial Herniation and Its Management* by Brian T. Andrews, MD and Lawrence H. Pitts, MD © 1991, Futura Publishing Co., Inc., Mount Kisco, NY.

additional patients have been treated with this protocol. In this chapter, we present our findings in the entire series of 153 patients and discuss the rationale for their treatment.

Protocol

The initial assessment, resuscitation, and emergency management have been described (see Chapters 3 and 4). Emergency burr-hole exploration was considered only if there was a clear history or external evidence of head trauma and clinical signs of transtentorial herniation or upper brain stem dysfunction. Patients were generally transported to the operating room within 20 minutes after admission. The head was shaved, sterilized with Betadine solution, and draped for bilateral surgical exploration (Fig. 7-1). The initial burr-hole was placed in the temporal region ipsilateral to the dilated pupil or, if both pupils were dilated, contralateral to the more severe hemiparesis or motor abnormalities. If both pupils were dilated and there were no localizing neurological deficits, the initial burr-hole was on the side of visible trauma or over the left (and presumed dominant) hemisphere. If the initial temporal craniectomy did not reveal an epidural

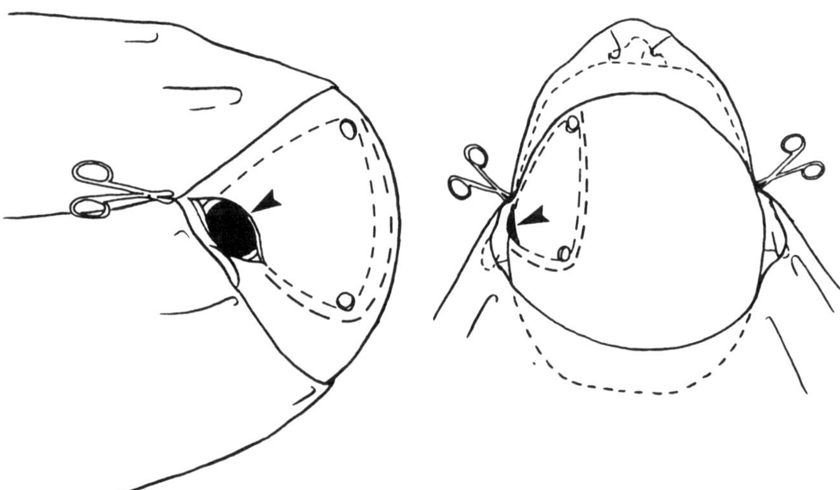

Figure 7-1. Side *(left)* and top *(right)* views showing the technique for draping the scalp to allow bilateral placement of frontal, temporal, and parietal burr-holes, and conversion of burr-holes to a large craniotomy, if needed. An epidural hematoma at the temporal burr-hole is shown *(arrowheads)*.

hematoma, the dura mater was incised and the subdural space was examined. If no lesion was found, a Betadine-soaked sponge was placed into the wound, and a temporal burr-hole was placed on the opposite side. A complete exploration consisted of bilateral temporal, frontal, and parietal burr-holes oriented for easy conversion to a large craniotomy (Fig. 7-2).

Epidural or subdural hematomas were considered significant if they were greater than 5 mm thick or present at more than one burr-hole site. Upon discovery of a significant hematoma, the exposure was immediately converted to a large craniotomy and the mass lesion was removed. Burr-holes were later placed over the opposite hemisphere because extra-axial mass lesions may be present bilaterally.[3] Before closure, an 8-French red rubber catheter was inserted into the subdural space or into a lateral ventricle and brought out through a small scalp incision for continuous monitoring of the ICP. Urgent general surgical procedures were usually performed during exploration; orthopedic and other procedures were deferred until after the neurosurgical operation.

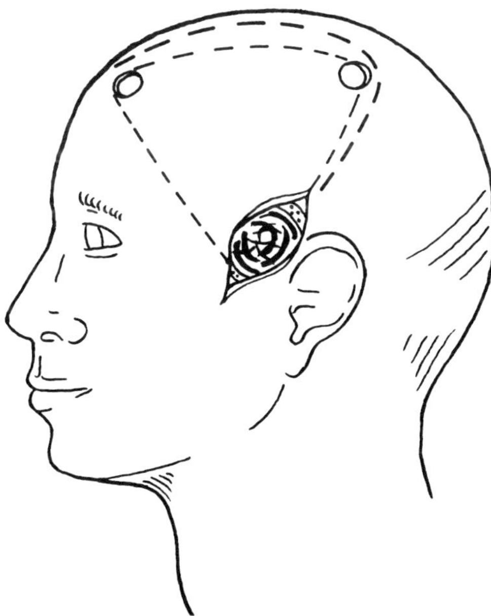

Figure 7-2. Burr-hole placement that allows for conversion to a large craniotomy for removal of an acute intracranial hematoma, if present.

Patients in whom intracranial hematomas were not identified surgically and whose cardiovascular status was stable were taken from the operating room to the computerized tomography (CT) suite. If the CT brain scans showed a significant intracranial hematoma, the patient was returned to the operating room for evacuation of the mass lesion. All patients were admitted from the operating room or CT scanner to the intensive care unit, where the ICP was monitored and aggressive attempts were made to control elevated ICP with a variety of techniques, including hyperventilation and hyperosmolar therapy. Their nutritional, metabolic, and infection status was closely monitored, and abnormalities were treated.

Summary of Cases

One hundred fifty-three patients are included in this analysis. There were 115 men and 38 women, with a mean age of 37 years (range 2–83 years). Fifty-three patients were injured in falls, 46 in vehicle-pedestrian accidents, 38 as motor vehicle occupants, and 11 in assaults; in five patients, the mechanism of injury was unknown. The clinical findings are summarized in Table 7-1.

Table 7-1 Clinical Findings at Admission in 153 Patients

Finding	*No. of Patients*
Cardiac arrest	10
Systemic hypotension (SBP < 80 mm Hg)	32
Single dilated pupil	95 (62%)
with hemiparesis/hemiplegia* or asymmetrical posturing	42
with symmetrical localizing or complex flexion	15
with flaccidity	38
Bilaterally dilated, fixed pupils	58 (38%)
with bilateral flexor posturing	13
with bilateral extensor posturing	15
with flaccidity	27
motor examination not recorded	3
Glasgow coma score (GCS)	
Median	4
Range	3–15
Progressive deterioration from GCS of 12–15 in the emergency room	8
GCS of 3	67
GCS of 4	28

*Contralateral to dilated pupil in 31 patients and ipsilateral in 10.

Surgical Findings

Exploratory burr-holes were positive in 93 patients (61%) and negative in 60 (39%) (Table 7-2). Subdural hematomas, detected unilaterally in 68 patients (73%) and bilaterally in 12 (12.9%), were the most common intracranial mass lesions. Epidural hematomas were detected unilaterally in seven patients (7.5%) and bilaterally in one. Unilateral intracerebral hematomas that required evacuation were detected along with a subdural hematoma in four patients. In one a small, deep-seated hematoma was identified by intraoperative ultrasonography but not evacuated. Depressed skull fractures were identified and treated in two patients. Patients with positive burr-hole findings were significantly older than those with negative findings (43.5 vs. 32 years, $p < 0.001$) and were most often injured in falls (41%) and vehicle-pedestrian accidents (31%). Motor vehicle accidents were the most common mechanism of injury in patients with negative findings (37%).

Among 95 patients admitted with anisocoria, 59 (62%) had a positive burr-hole exploration, which was ipsilateral to the dilated pupil in 54 (91.5%) and contralateral in five (8.5%). The percentage of positive burr-holes in this group was not influenced by the presence of systemic hypotension. Among patients with bilaterally dilated, fixed pupils, however, positive burr-holes were less common in patients with systemic hypotension or initial cardiac arrest than in those without such findings (36% vs. 58%).

Table 7-2 Surgical Findings in 153 Patients

Finding	*No. of Patients*
Positive burr-hole exploration	93 (61%)
Unilateral	
Subdural hematoma	68 (73%)
Epidural hematoma	7 (7.5%)
Subdural and intracerebral hematoma	4 (4.3%)
Intracerebral hematoma (detected by intraoperative ultrasonography)	1
Bilateral	
Subdural hematomas	12 (12.9%)
Epidural hematomas	1
Depressed skull fracture	2
Negative burr-hole exploration	60 (39%)
Complete exploration	48
Incomplete exploration	12

Table 7-3 Surgically Significant Hematomas Not Detected by Burr-Hole Exploration

Hematoma Location	*No. of Patients*
Subdural	6
Incomplete exploration	5
Contralateral to a positive exploration	1
Epidural (contralateral to a positive exploration)	1
Intracerebral	6
Undetected by intraoperative ultrasonography	3

Hematomas that required surgical removal were not detected by burr-hole exploration in 13 patients (Table 7-3). CT scanning or autopsy showed a residual or missed extra-axial hematoma on the side of an *incomplete* burr-hole exploration in five patients; in each case the mass was located away from the initial burr-holes. In two patients, hematomas were missed because burr-holes placed were not placed on the opposite side after evacuation of a mass. Six patients (4%) had intracerebral hematomas that were not detected surgically; in two of these patients, however, a subdural hematoma had been identified and evacuated. In three recent patients, intracerebral hematomas were identified by CT scanning after bilateral intraoperative real-time ultrasonography failed to show intra-axial lesions. These hematomas were either missed by ultrasound examination or developed after the initial exploration but before postoperative CT scanning. Each of the intracerebral hematomas required subsequent surgical removal.

Outcome

The outcome was determined with the Glasgow Outcome Scale[14] after a mean follow-up of 11 months (range 1–37 months) (Table 7-4). Fourteen patients (9%) had a good recovery (little or no physical impairment), 14 were moderately disabled, 15 were severely disabled, and one was vegetative. One hundred four patients (68%) died, most within 1 week after injury. The outcome of five patients is unknown.

The findings in patients who had a good recovery are shown in

Table 7-4 Outcome in 153 Patients

Outcome	*No. of Patients*
Good recovery	14 (9%)
Moderate disability	14
Severe disability	15
Vegetative	1
Dead	104 (68%)
Within 8 hours of admission	36
Within 7 days of injury	36
After 7 days	32
Unknown	5

Table 7-5. Their mean age was slightly less than the average for the series (34 vs. 37 years), but three were older than 65 years. Their initial mean Glasgow coma score (GCS) was higher than that of the entire series (8 vs. 4); four patients who had an initial GCS of 12 or greater deteriorated abruptly in the emergency room. No patient was in cardiac arrest, hypotensive, or had bilaterally dilated, unresponsive pupils at admission. Nine patients had a hemiparesis. Seven of the eight patients (57%) with positive surgical findings had a unilateral subdural hematoma and one had an epidural hematoma. Postoperative CT scans showed no missed hematomas. One comatose patient in whom burr-hole exploration showed normal, pulsatile

Table 7-5 Clinical Findings in 28 Patients Who Had Good Outcome or Were Moderately Disabled

Variable	*Good Outcome*	*Moderate Disability*
Number of patients	14	14
Age (years)		
Mean	34	29
Range	2–74	9–56
Anisocoria	14 (100%)	12 (86%)
Hemiparesis	9 (64%)	4
Symmetrical localizing or complex flexion	3	2
Extensor posturing	1	5
Flaccid	1	3
Glasgow Coma Score		
Mean	8	6
Range	3–15	3–15
Deteriorated abruptly	4	1
Positive burr-hole exploration	8 (57%)	7 (50%)

brain had an abnormally dilated pupil as a result of childhood eye trauma. This patient had false-positive clinical signs of transtentorial herniation.

Patients who were moderately disabled were also younger than the mean age for the series (29 vs. 37 years) and had a higher initial mean GCS (6 vs. 4) (Table 7-5). No patient was admitted in cardiac arrest; two were hypotensive and two had bilaterally dilated, unresponsive pupils. Only four patients had a hemiparesis. Surgical exploration disclosed subdural hematomas in six patients (bilaterally in one) and an epidural hematoma in one. Postoperative CT scans showed no missed lesions.

Among 95 patients with anisocoria, 62% had positive burr-hole exploration and 27% had a good outcome or were moderately disabled. Among the 58 patients with bilaterally dilated, fixed pupils, 59% had a positive exploration, but only 3.5% had a good outcome or were moderately disabled. The difference in functional outcome between these two groups was significant ($p < 0.05$). Among the 28 patients with bilaterally dilated, fixed pupils who were resuscitated from cardiac arrest or were admitted with systemic hypotension, only 36% had an intracranial mass detected, and all died. Overall, 40 of 42 patients with initial cardiac arrest or systemic hypotension died or were left severely disabled or vegetative.

Rationale

Although clinical signs of transtentorial herniation occasionally indicate a primary brain stem injury,[10,14] patients with clinical signs of brain stem dysfunction have a high incidence of intracranial hematomas, most of which are extra-axial and can therefore be detected by burr-hole exploration.[3–5,7,9,10,13,15] Prompt removal of such lesions can relieve brain stem compression and minimize injury caused by displacement of the brain and by elevated ICP.[3,17,23,26,27,29] The principal argument for surgical exploration before CT scanning is to speed the diagnosis and evacuation of the mass lesion. Our patients generally arrived in the emergency room within 1 hour after injury and were transported to the operating room within 20 minutes. Ninety-nine (65%) of them had significant extra-axial hematomas that were potentially detectable by complete bilateral burr-hole exploration.

Patients with brain stem dysfunction and expanding mass lesions do best if treated soon after injury.[9,25–27] Seelig et al.[27] reported that 12 of 61 patients with severe traumatic brain stem dysfunction survived, but only the six patients in whom a subdural hematoma was evacuated within 2½ hours of injury had a good outcome or moderate disability. Mahoney et al.[17] found that only three of 41 patients with progressive signs of transtentorial herniation after trauma had a good outcome. All three had an immediate clinical response to emergency burr-hole placement and evacuation of a hematoma. Among 52 patients with traumatic intracranial hematomas and decerebrate posturing, Gutterman and Shenken[9] reported that nine of 15 who had surgical evacuation within 4 hours of injury suffered only mild residual neurological deficits. Only two of five patients treated surgically within 6 hours survived, both with severe deficits, and all patients treated more than 6 hours after injury died.

CT scanning is clearly indicated for patients with altered consciousness and intact brain stem reflexes after severe head injury and is invaluable for evaluating patients without a clear history of trauma, regardless of the presence of brain stem dysfunction. Obtaining a CT scan, however, takes time. In one series, the mean time from deterioration to coma to the start of surgery in 10 patients in whom CT scans showed a mass lesion was 1 hour and 20 minutes.[23] While the CT scans are being obtained, there is continued mechanical compression of the brain stem. Moreover, the patient is relatively isolated inside the scanner, which interrupts continuous intensive monitoring and makes it difficult to perform serial clinical evaluations and to diagnose and treat systemic complications, such as hypotension and cardiac arrhythmias.

In contrast, direct admission to the operating room for burr-hole exploration avoids the delay inherent in CT scanning, allows continuous intensive monitoring, and enables systemic injuries and medical complications to be detected and treated immediately. If the exploration is positive, the lesion can be evacuated immediately. If the exploration is negative, intracranial pressure can be monitored; systemic injuries have been treated and stabilized and the patient can safely undergo CT scanning. The morbidity of burr-hole placement is negligible.

A complete bilateral exploration consisting of frontal, temporal, and parietal burr-holes is necessary to accurately detect extra-axial hematomas. In our initial review of 100 patients,[3] significant subdural and epidural hematomas were missed in six cases due to an incomplete exploration; among the subsequent 53 patients only one subdural hematoma was missed for that reason. No extra-axial hematoma was missed in patients who had a complete bilateral burr-hole exploration. Intracerebral hematomas were missed at surgery in three of the initial 100 patients; in two, burr-hole exploration had shown an overlying subdural hematoma, which was promptly evacuated.

Since 1985, we have used intraoperative bilateral ultrasound imaging of the brain to detect intraparenchymal mass lesions. In five cases, intracerebral hematomas were detected; in three others, ultrasonography was negative but postoperative CT scanning showed an intracerebral hematoma. Those lesions either were missed by ultrasound imaging or developed subsequently from cerebral contusions. We have recently attempted to limit surgical exploration to one side only by performing intraoperative real-time ultrasonography of the whole brain and contralateral convexity through unilateral burr-holes (see Chapter 9). The results are encouraging but remain preliminary.

Among the first 100 patients in our series,[3] extracerebral hematomas were more common in older patients and after falls and assaults than after high-speed motor vehicle accidents, which tended to cause diffuse injury. The mean age of patients with negative burr-hole exploration and negative CT scans was significantly less than that of patients with mass lesions (35 vs. 45.3 years, $p < 0.001$). Burr-hole exploration was positive in 36% of patients younger than 30 years of age, compared with 60% of those 30 to 59 years old and 75% of those 60 years and older ($p < 0.025$).[3] We therefore began to exclude from the surgical protocol young adults injured in motor vehicle accidents unless they showed clinical signs of *deterioration* to coma and signs of *progressive* brain stem compression; as many as 76% of such patients have a significant intracranial hematoma.[24] (Children younger than 18 years of age with brain stem dysfunction after head injury have a significant incidence of hematomas and therefore undergo burr-hole exploration unless they are severely hypotensive.) Patients with initial cardiac arrest or severe systemic hypotension (systolic blood pressure below 60 mm Hg) also have a low incidence of intracranial mass lesions[2] and therefore are excluded unless they required immediate surgery for life-threatening systemic injuries. Since these exclusions were instituted in 1986, the percentage of positive burr-hole explorations has increased to 55% of patients 18 to 30 years old, 75% of those ages 30 to 59, and 89% of those 60 years and older. Overall, 37 (70%) of the 53 patients treated since 1986 have had positive burr-holes; four had bilateral mass lesions, and two had a significant intracerebral hematoma in addition to a subdural hematoma.

Among patients with anisocoria and a significant intracranial hematoma, the mass was ipsilateral to the dilated pupil in 91.5% of cases and contralateral in 8.5%. Previous reports[3,21] have also suggested that a traumatic intracranial mass is most often ipsilateral to the dilated pupil. Hemiparesis is less useful in localizing the side of a mass lesion in patients with Kernohan's notch phenomenon.

Although traumatic transtentorial herniation carries a poor prognosis,[3,9,10,12,22,26,27] a gratifying number of patients may have a functional recovery. Overall, 9% of our 153 patients had a good outcome and 9% were only moderately disabled. Compared with patients who died or were severely disabled or vegetative, these patients were generally younger, had a higher initial GCS, and had anisocoria. In other series, younger age[4,9,16,20,30] and a higher initial GCS[1,2,26] have been associated with a better prognosis for recovery. Among patients who had a good outcome, 57% had a unilateral subdural or epidural hematoma. Among those having a moderate disability, 50% had a mass lesion which was evacuated. In our original series[3] only 44% of the patients in these groups harbored a significant intracranial hematoma. Clearly, some patients with a primary injury of the brain stem may do well with supportive care.

Bilaterally dilated, fixed pupils indicate a dismal prognosis.[4,16,18,20,27,29] Only 3.5% of our patients with that finding had a good outcome or were moderately disabled, compared with 27% of those with anisocoria. Stone et al.[29] found that 25% of patients with a single dilated pupil ipsilateral to a subdural hematoma had a functional recovery, compared with only 11% of those with bilaterally absent pupillary function. In the series of Seelig et al.,[27] only 10% of patients with severe upper brain stem dysfunction after head injury had a good outcome or moderate disability.

We do not intend to suggest or to imply that burr-hole exploration should replace CT scanning in the initial evaluation of all severely head-injured patients. CT scans are invaluable in assessing head injury patients who are lethargic or comatose but have intact brain stem function. However, CT scans obtained shortly after injury may fail to show a small but enlarging extracranial mass or cerebral contusion that may evolve into an intracerebral hematoma requiring evacuation.[3] Thus, CT scans or diagnostic burr-hole exploration soon after injury may not detect lesions that eventually require surgery.

Given the high incidence of expanding extra-axial hematomas and the potential morbidity of additional delay in diagnosis and evacuation of such lesions, emergency burr-hole exploration before CT scanning is a reasonable and justified approach to the management of severely head-injured patients with signs of brain stem dysfunction.[3,4,6,9–11,17,27] We cannot say that burr-hole exploration improves upon the survival and recovery rates of patients who undergo preoperative CT scanning. To demonstrate this would require a prospective, randomized study comparing the two techniques. Our results do confirm the high incidence of extra-axial hematomas in patients with traumatic transtentorial herniation, especially those older than 30 years of age. In adults 18 to 30 years of age without *progressive* signs of brain stem dysfunction and in those with severe hypotension or initial cardiac arrest, exploratory burr-holes are often negative.[2,3] In such cases, management decisions should be based on the results of CT scanning, if possible.

References

1. Andrews BT: Management of delayed posttraumatic intracerebral hemorrhage. Contemp Neurosurg 10:1-6, 1988.
2. Andrews BT, Levy ML, Pitts LH: The implications of systemic hypotension for the neurological examination in patients with severe head injury. Surg Neurol 28:419-422, 1987.
3. Andrews BT, Pitts LH, Lovely MP, et al.: Is computed tomographic scanning necessary in patients with tentorial herniation? Results of immediate surgical exploration without computed tomography in 100 patients. Neurosurgery 19:408-414, 1986.
4. Becker DP, Miller JD, Ward JD, et al.: The outcome from severe head injury with early diagnosis and intensive management. J Neurosurg 47:491-502, 1977.
5. Bowers SA, Marshall LF: Outcome in 200 consecutive cases of severe head injury treated in San Diego County: a prospective analysis. Neurosurgery 6:237-241, 1980.

6. Brender SJ, Selverstone B: Recovery from decerebration. Brain 93:381-392, 1970.
7. Gennarelli TA, Spielman GM, Langfitt TW, et al.: Influence of the type of intracranial lesion on outcome from severe head injury–a multicenter study using a new classification system. J Neurosurg 56:26-32, 1982.
8. Grossman R: Treatment of patients with intracranial hematomas. N Engl J Med 304:1540-1541, 1981.
9. Gutterman P, Shenken HA: Prognostic features in recovery from decerebration. J Neurosurg 32:330-335, 1979.
10. Hoff JT, Spetzler R, Winestock D: Head injury and early signs of tentorial herniation–a management dilemma. West J Med 128: 112-116, 1978.
11. Howell DA: Upper brain stem compression and foraminal impaction with intracranial space-occupying lesions and brain swelling. Brain 82:525-550, 1959.
12. Jamieson KG, Yelland JD: Surgically treated traumatic subdural hematomas. J Neurosurg 37:137-149, 1972.
13. Jamieson KG, Yelland JD: Traumatic intracerebral hematoma. Report of 63 surgically treated cases. J Neurosurg 37:528-532, 1972.
14. Jennett B, Bond M: Assessment of outcome after severe brain damage. Lancet 1:480-484, 1975.
15. Jennett B, Teasdale G: Management of Head Injuries. Philadelphia, PA: FA Davis, 1981.
16. Jennett B, Teasdale G, Braakman R, et al.: Prognosis of patients with severe head injury. Neurosurgery 4:283-289, 1979.
17. Mahoney BD, Rockswold GL, Ruiz E, et al.: Emergency twist-drill trephination. Neurosurgery 8:551-554, 1981.
18. Marshall LF, Barba D, Toole BM, et al.: Oval pupil: clinical significance and relationship to intracranial hypertension. J Neurosurg 58:566-568, 1983.
19. Ogsbury JS, Schneck SA, Lehman RA: Aspects of interhemispheric subdural hematoma, including falx syndrome. J Neurol Neurosurg Psychiatry 41:72-75, 1978.
20. Overgaard J, Christensen S, Hvid-Hansen O, et al.: Prognosis after head injury based on early clinical examination. Lancet 2:7830-7835, 1973.
21. Pitts LH: Neurological evaluation of the head injured patient. Clin Neurosurg 29:203-224, 1981.

22. Richards T, Hoff J: Factors affecting survival from acute subdural hematoma. Surgery 75:253-258, 1974.
23. Rockswold GL: Reply to letter: Management of closed head injury patients who "talked and deteriorated." Neurosurgery 22: 614, 1988.
24. Rockswold GL, Leonard PR, Nagib MG: Analysis of management in thirty-three closed head injury patients who "talked and deteriorated." Neurosurgery 21:51-55, 1987.
25. Sachs E, Bernat JM: Recovery from acute subdural hematoma and uncal herniation due to ruptured intracranial aneurysm. Neurosurgery 3:66-67, 1978.
26. Seelig JM, Becker DP, Miller JD, et al.: Traumatic acute subdural hematoma. Major mortality reduction in comatose patients treated within four hours. N Engl J Med 304:1511-1517, 1981.
27. Seelig JM, Greenberg RP, Becker DP, et al.: Reversible brain stem dysfunction following acute traumatic subdural hematoma–a clinical and electrophysiological study. J Neurosurg 55:516-523, 1981.
28. Soloniuk D, Pitts LH, Lovely MP, et al.: Traumatic intracerebral hematomas: timing of appearance and indications for operative removal. J Trauma 26:787-793, 1986.
29. Stone JL, Rifai MHS, Surgar O, et al.: Subdural hematomas. I. Acute subdural hematoma: progress in definition, clinical pathology and therapy. Surg Neurol 19:216-231, 1983.
30. Teasdale G, Skene A, Parker L, et al: Age and outcome of severe head injury. Acta Neurochir Suppl 28(Wien):140-143, 1979.

CHAPTER 8

Traumatic Intracerebral Hematomas: Formation and Effect of Location on the Occurrence of Transtentorial Herniation

Intracerebral hematomas are common after head injury but usually develop several hours to days or even longer after the traumatic event.[1,9,26] As a result, these lesions are of less immediate concern than extra-axial hematomas in severely head-injured patients. However, traumatic intracerebral hematomas can develop immediately; those in the temporal region are especially likely to cause brain stem compression resulting in transtentorial herniation.[2]

Intracerebral Hemorrhage Formation After Trauma

Acute and delayed hemorrhages within the brain, although less common than epidural and subdural hematomas, are a well-known problem after head injury. Knowledge of the factors that cause these lesions is important because early recognition and prompt management are essential for optimal outcome. Awareness of the time course of their formation is essential in order to maintain a high level of suspicion during the period when intracerebral hematomas are likely to occur.

Recognition of intracerebral hematomas within the first 24 hours used to be considered extremely uncommon,[5,7] being much

From *Traumatic Transtentorial Herniation and Its Management* by Brian T. Andrews, MD and Lawrence H. Pitts, MD © 1991, Futura Publishing Co., Inc., Mount Kisco, NY.

more frequent in subsequent days or longer afterward.[1,9,10–12,25] The introduction of CT led to more accurate recognition of early hematomas and better understanding of the timing of their formation after head injury. In 1985, Soloniuk et al.[26] reported that 20% of significant intracerebral hemorrhages in patients with severe head injury were identified on computed tomography (CT) scans at admission to the hospital. Another 7% of the lesions requiring surgery were recognized during the first 6 hours after admission, and a total of 35% developed within the first 24 hours; 46% were detected 24 to 72 hours and 20% more than 72 hours after injury. One hematoma was surgically evacuated 20 days after injury. Similarly, Gudeman et al.[10] found that 33% of traumatic intracerebral hemorrhages were diagnosed during the first 24 hours and 66% within 48 hours after admission. One hematoma (8%) developed 24 days after head injury. Numerous other reports have confirmed that intracerebral hemorrhages are relatively rare immediately after head injury but may occur days, weeks, or even months later.[1]

Among severely head-injured patients admitted with clinical signs of transtentorial herniation, acute intracerebral hematomas are also relatively rare. Andrews et al.[3] found that among 100 such patients only three had acute intracerebral hematomas, whereas 62% had epidural or subdural hematomas. In a more recent series of 17 children with initial signs of transtentorial herniation, only one (6%) had a small intracerebral hematoma, which was diagnosed soon after admission.[4]

The Effect of Hematoma Location on the Occurrence of Transtentorial Herniation

Intracerebral hematomas usually cause focal neurological deficits and, if large enough, may alter the level of consciousness as well.[8,13–15,20,24,26] Through their mass effect, such lesions may in rare cases compress the upper brain stem, resulting in the clinical triad of transtentorial herniation.[6,8] Brain stem compression and loss of consciousness markedly worsen the prognosis, regardless of treatment.[6,8,16,20,23] Many authors have cautioned that cerebellar hematomas may rapidly lead to brain stem compression and that prompt surgical removal is usually warranted.[6,8,16,17,20,21,23] This concern has not, however, extended to supratentorial hematomas. Nevertheless, in recent years Marshall[15] has found that patients with mass lesions in the temporal lobe after trauma were at significant risk for brain stem compression and that such compression could occur without a detectable rise in intracranial pressure (ICP).

A recent study from our institution has also shown that traumatic hematomas of the temporal lobe are much more likely to cause transtentorial herniation than are other supratentorial hematomas.[2] In that study, we reviewed the course of 45 patients who had supratentorial intracerebral hemorrhages localized primarily to a single lobe of the brain.[2] CT scans were obtained at admission or at the time of significant clinical deterioration. The volume of the hematoma was estimated by calculating the product of the anteroposterior, medial-lateral, and supero-inferior diameters of the lesion on axial CT scans. The maximal midline shift was also measured.

The patients—34 men and 11 women, aged 6 to 89 years (mean 47 years)—were separated into three groups according to the location of the hematoma. The lesions were frontal in 18 patients (Fig. 8-1), temporal or temporoparietal in 17 (Fig. 8-2), and parieto-occipital in 10. The hematomas were caused by head trauma in 32 patients, hypertension in five, bacterial endocarditis in two, embolic events in two, and aneurysm rupture in one. In three patients, the cause of hemorrhage was unknown despite cerebral arteriography. The three groups were well matched for age, mechanism of injury, initial Glasgow coma score, and frequency of hemiparesis (Table 8-1).

No patient with a frontal or parieto-occipital hematoma had abnormal brain stem reflexes or the clinical triad of transtentorial herniation. In contrast, ipsilateral signs of transtentorial herniation were present at admission in three of 18 patients with temporal or temporoparietal hematomas and developed within 12 hours in four others ($p < 0.05$). The hematoma was the result of head injury in six of the seven patients.

The mean volume of temporal and temporoparietal hematomas (41 ± 21 cc) was not significantly different from that of frontal (47 ± 28 cc) or parieto-occipital hematomas (53 ± 26 cc). None of the six patients with temporal hematomas 30 cc or smaller had signs of brain stem compression early in their hospital course, whereas seven of the 11 patients with temporal hematomas larger than 30 cc developed signs of transtentorial herniation ($p < 0.05$). The size of the lesion correlated strongly with the maximal midline shift in patients

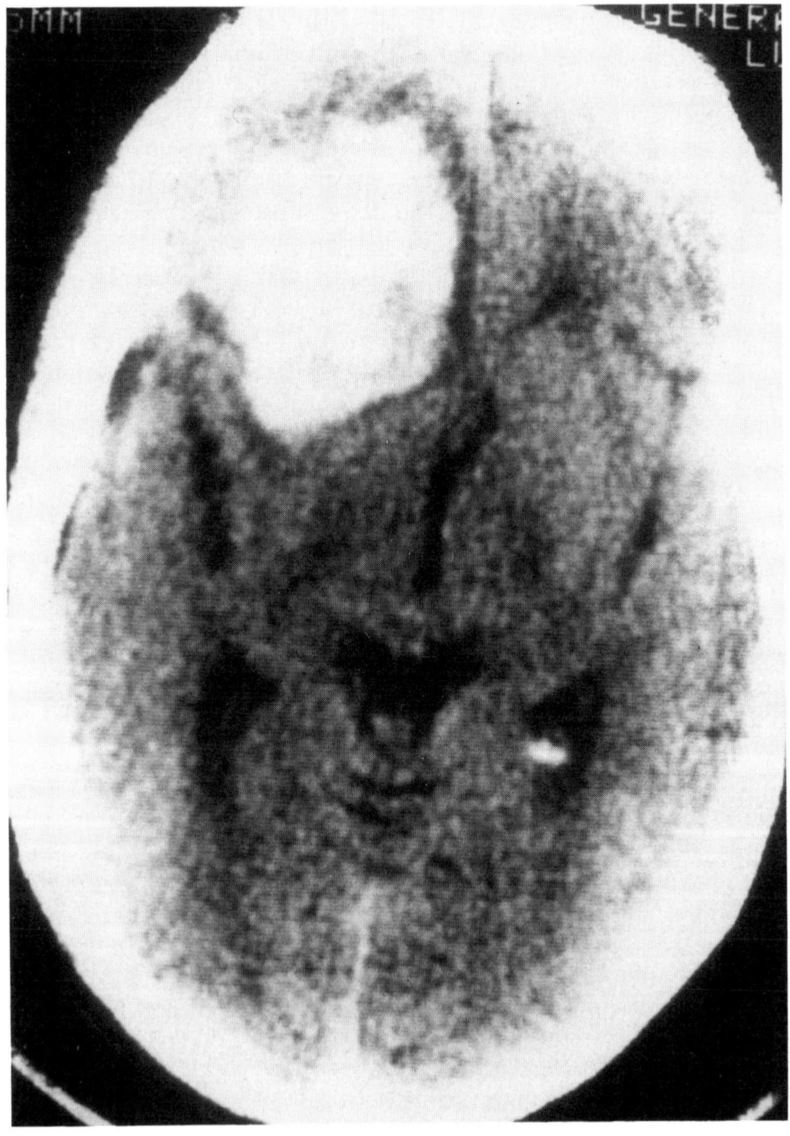

Figure 8-1. Noncontrast CT scan showing a frontal lobe hematoma.

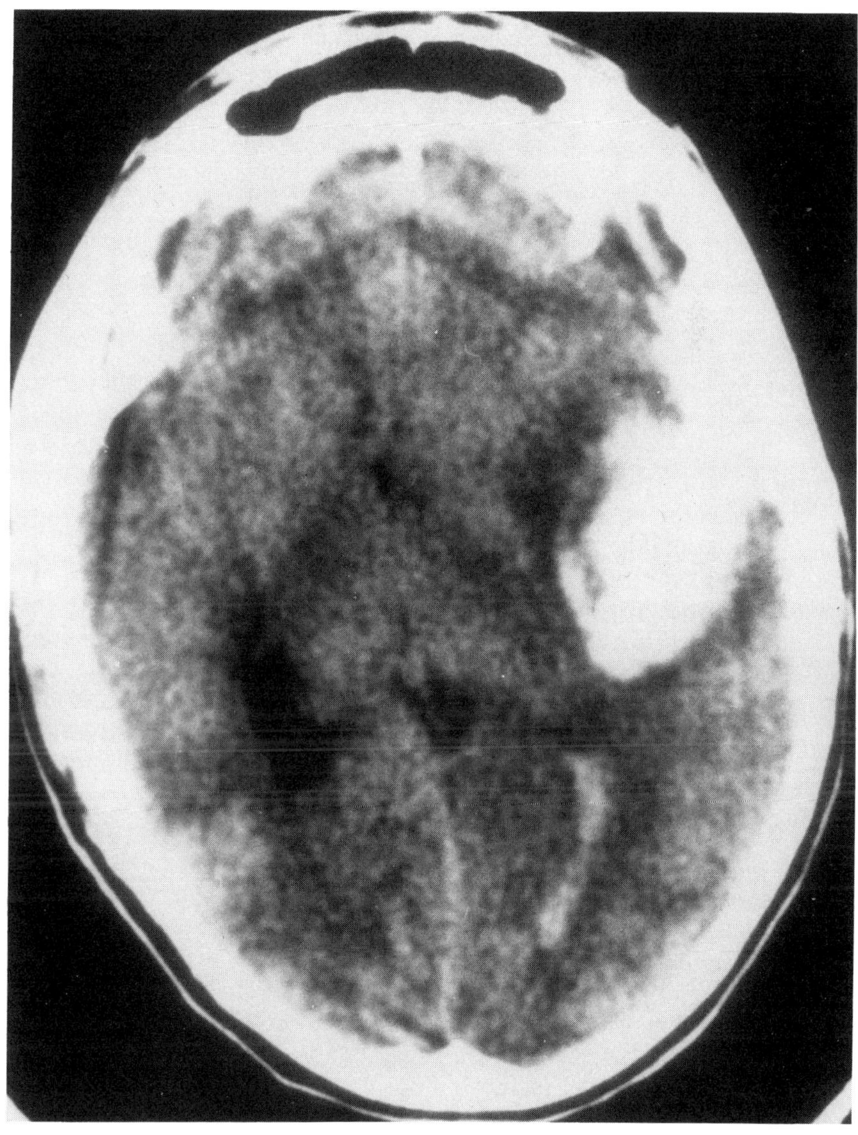

Figure 8-2. Noncontrast CT scan showing a temporal lobe hematoma.

Table 8-1 Clinical Findings at Presentation in 45 Patients with Supratentorial Hematoma*

		Glasgow Coma Score		
Hematoma Location	*No. Cases*	*> 8*	*≤ 8*	*Hemiparesis*
Frontal	18	14 (78%)	4 (22%)	6 (33%)
Parieto-occipital	10	9 (90%)	1 (10%)	3 (30%)
Temporal/temporoparietal	17	15 (88%)	2 (12%)	3 (18%)

*Reproduced with permission from Andrews BT et al.: The effect of intracerebral hematoma location on the risk of brain-stem compression and on clinical outcome. J Neurosurg 69:518-522, 1988.

with temporal or temporoparietal hematomas (r = 0.829), but not in those with frontal (r = 0.426) or parieto-occipital (r = 0.24) lesions.

Craniotomy was performed to evacuate the mass in eight of 18 patients with frontal hematomas, four of 10 with parieto-occipital hematomas (one case was urgent), and nine of 17 with temporal and temporoparietal hematomas. Two of the three patients with clinical signs of transtentorial herniation at admission immediately underwent a craniotomy. The third patient, who had anisocoria with bilaterally reactive pupils, a mild hemiparesis, and changes in mental status, had a very small temporal hematoma (31.5 cc) and was treated successfully with mannitol and dehydration. In each of the four patients who developed signs of transtentorial herniation within 12 hours after admission, CT scans showed a temporal hematoma, which was immediately evacuated.

The neurological outcome[12] was much worse among patients with temporal or temporoparietal hematomas than among those in the other two groups (Table 8-2). Only three of 17 patients (18%) with temporal hematomas had a good outcome, compared with 44% of those with frontal and 60% of those with parieto-occipital hematomas (both $p < 0.05$ vs. temporal group). None of the patients with signs of transtentorial herniation had a good outcome: two were moderately disabled, two were severely disabled, and three (43%) died. All eight deaths in the temporal and temporoparietal group, but only two of four in the frontal group and none of four in the parieto-occipital group, resulted from the effects of the hematoma itself.

The indications for removal of post-traumatic hematomas include a depressed level of consciousness, a focal neurological deficit

Table 8-2 Outcome at Discharge According to Hematoma Location*

			Temporal	
Outcome	*Frontal*	*Parieto-occipital*	*Total*	*With Herniation*
Good	8 (44%)	6 (60%)	3 (18%)	0 (0%)
Moderately disabled	3	0	7	2
Severely disabled	3	0	2	2
Dead	4 (22%)	4 (40%)	5 (29%)	3 (43%)
Total	18	10	17	7

*Reproduced with permission from Andrews BT et al.: The effect of intracerebral hematoma location on the risk of brain-stem compression and on clinical outcome. J Neurosurg 69:518-522, 1988.

associated with a hematoma in an anatomically appropriate area,[6] a deteriorating or unimproving neurological status,[19,26] intractable elevation of ICP,[6,26] and a significant midline shift on CT scan.[26] To that list we would add the clinical signs of transtentorial herniation associated with a hematoma in the temporal lobe.[2]

Cerebellar hematomas have been considered treacherous lesions, especially those larger than 3 cm in diameter or 30 cc in volume, because they may lead rapidly and often irreversibly to brain stem dysfunction.[6,20,23] It has often been recommended that such hematomas be removed, even when signs of brain stem compression have not yet developed.[6,20,23] Until recently, similar recommendations had not been made for supratentorial hematomas.[2,15]

In our series, patients with traumatic temporal or temporoparietal hematomas were more likely to develop transtentorial herniation than those with frontal or parieto-occipital hematomas of similar volume (41% vs. 0%),[2] and therefore had a significantly worse outcome. Temporal hematomas probably cause mechanical compression of the upper brain stem because they are contained within the middle fossa anteriorly, laterally, and inferiorly and by a large mass of brain parenchyma superiorly and posteriorly. Therefore, the path of least resistance may be medial, toward the ambient cistern and the brain stem. In addition, the temporal lobe is adjacent to the upper brain stem, whereas the frontal and parieto-occipital lobes are much more distant. Finally, while the relatively rigid falx cerebri may prevent or limit an acute midline shift caused by a frontal or parieto-occipital hematoma, no such barrier exists for temporal hematomas. This premise is supported by the finding that hematoma size correlated strongly with midline shift in patients with temporal and temporoparietal hematomas but not in those with hematomas in the other two regions.

Marshall et al.[15] have reported that temporal hematomas could cause pupillary abnormalities consistent with transtentorial herniation (so-called oval pupil) despite a normal ICP (up to 20 mm Hg). Pupillary abnormalities did not occur until the ICP exceeded 35 mm Hg in patients with parietal mass lesions and 40 mm Hg in those with diffuse brain swelling. The oval pupil frequently returned to normal when the ICP was reduced by medical or surgical means. A recent study of cats subjected to balloon inflation in the temporal lobe showed that pressure increased in the temporal lobe and midbrain without a generalized increase in ICP measured in the frontal lobe. These results suggest that monitoring the ICP may not be adequate for predicting (and thus preventing) the development of transtentorial herniation when a hematoma is present within the temporal lobe.

Transtentorial herniation occurred in our study *only* among patients with temporal hematomas larger than 30 cc,[2] nearly two-thirds of whom developed brain stem compression. Coincidentally, previous reports have suggested that cerebellar hematomas larger than 30 cc are particularly likely to cause brain stem compression.[2,16,19,23] We therefore recommend that temporal and temporoparietal hematomas larger than 30 cc be promptly evacuated to avoid the development of transtentorial herniation.

Head injury was the cause of the hematoma in six of the seven patients in our series who developed signs of brain stem compression.[2] This may simply reflect the predominance of head-injured patients in this group or may indicate that intracerebral hematomas due to trauma are more likely than those of other causes to enlarge and compress the brain stem. Transtentorial herniation is uncommon among patients with spontaneous hemorrhage in the temporal lobe or in other supratentorial regions.[13,24] The overall mortality rate after spontaneous lobar hemorrhage has been reported to be 11.5%–21%.[13,22,24] In one study,[26] traumatic temporal hematomas proved fatal more often than hematomas in other sites (57% vs. 37%). Although no association between hematoma location and brain stem compression was established in that study, the high mortality rate among our patients with temporal hematomas (29%) was specifically due to the poor outcome of the patients with signs of brain stem compression.

In summary, the majority of traumatic intracerebral hematomas occur hours to days after injury. However, acute and immediate intracerebral hematomas do occur, and those in the temporal or temporoparietal region are much more likely to cause early and often rapid development of clinical signs of transtentorial herniation than hematomas in other locations. Temporal hematomas larger than 30 cc as estimated from CT scans are particularly likely to cause brain stem compression and should therefore be promptly evacuated.

References

1. Andrews BT: Management of delayed post-traumatic intracerebral hemorrhage. Contemp Neurosurg 10:1-6, 1988.
2. Andrews BT, Chiles BW, Olsen WL, et al.: The effect of intracerebral hematoma location on the risk of brain-stem compression and on clinical outcome. J Neurosurg 69:518-522, 1988.
3. Andrews BT, Pitts LH, Lovely MP, et al.: Is computed tomographic scanning necessary in patients with tentorial herniation? Results of immediate surgical exploration without computerized tomography in 100 patients. Neurosurgery 19: 408-414, 1986.
4. Andrews BT, Ross A, Pitts LH: The results of immediate exploratory burr-hole placement in children with post-traumatic transtentorial herniation. Surg Neurol 32:434-438, 1989.
5. Brown F, Mullen S, Duda E: Delayed traumatic intracerebral hematomas. J Neurosurg 48:1019-1022, 1978.
6. Cooper PR: Post-traumatic intracranial mass lesions. In Cooper PR (ed): Head Injury. 2nd ed. Baltimore, MD: Williams and Wilkins, 1987, pp 238-284.
7. Diaz FG, Yock DH, Larson D, et al.: Early diagnosis of delayed post-traumatic intracerebral hematomas. J Neurosurg 50: 217-223, 1979.
8. Fisher CM, Picard EH, Polak A, et al.: Acute hypertensive cerebellar hemorrhage: diagnosis and surgical treatment. J Nerv Ment Dis 140:38-57, 1965.
9. Fukamachi A, Nagaseki Y, Kohno K, et al.: The incidence and developmental process of delayed traumatic intracerebral haematomas. Acta Neurochir 74:35-39, 1985.

10. Gudeman S, Kishore P, Miller J, et al.: The genesis and significance of delayed traumatic intracerebral hematoma. Neurosurgery 5:309-313, 1979.
11. Hirsh L: Delayed traumatic intracerebral hematoma after surgical decompression. Neurosurgery 5:653-655, 1979.
12. Jennett B, Bond M: Assessment of outcome after severe brain damage: a practical scale. Lancet 1:480-484, 1975.
13. Kase CS, Williams JP, Wyatt DA, et al.: Lobar intracerebral hematomas: clinical and CT analysis of 22 cases. Neurology 32: 1146-1150, 1982.
14. Luessenhop AJ, Shevlin WA, Ferrero AA, et al.: Surgical management of primary intracerebral hemorrhage. J Neurosurg 27: 419-427, 1967.
15. Marshall LF, Cotten JM, Bowers-Marshall S, et al.: Pupillary abnormalities, elevated intracranial pressure and mass lesion location. In Miller JD, Teasdale GM, Rowan JO, et al. (eds): Intracranial Pressure VI. Berlin: Springer-Verlag, 1986.
16. McKissock W, Richardson A, Walsh L: Spontaneous cerebellar hemorrhage. A study of 34 consecutive cases treated surgically. Brain 83:1-9, 1960.
17. Melamed N, Satya-Murti S: Cerebellar hemorrhage. A review and reappraisal of benign cases. Arch Neurol 41:425-428, 1984.
18. Miller JD, Holaday HR, Peeler DF: Intracranial pressure changes from a temporal lobe mass in cats. Read before the Seventh International Symposium on Intracranial Pressure and Brain Injury, Ann Arbor, MI, June 19-23, 1988.
19. Morin MA, Pitts FW: Delayed apoplexy following head injury ("traumatische Spät-Apoplexie"). J Neurosurg 33:542-547, 1970.
20. Ojemann RG, Heros RC: Spontaneous brain hemorrhage. Stroke 14:468-475, 1983.
21. Ott KH, Kase CS, Ojemann RG, et al.: Cerebellar hemorrhage: diagnosis and treatment: a review of 56 cases. Arch Neurol 31: 160-167, 1974.
22. Paillas JE, Alliez B: Surgical treatment of spontaneous intracerebral hemorrhage: immediate and long-term results in 250 cases. J Neurosurg 39:145-151, 1973.
23. Pozzati E, Piazza G, Padovani R, et al.: Benign traumatic intracerebellar hematoma. Neurosurgery 8:102-103, 1981.
24. Ropper AH, Davis KR: Lobar cerebral hemorrhages: acute clinical syndromes in 26 cases. Ann Neurol 8:141-147, 1980.

25. Shallat R, Taekman M, Nagel R: Delayed complications of craniocerebral trauma: case report. Neurosurgery 8:569-573, 1981.
26. Soloniuk D, Pitts LH, Lovely M, et al.: Traumatic intracerebral hematomas: timing of appearance and indications for operative removal. J Trauma 26:787-793, 1986.

CHAPTER 9

Use of Intraoperative Ultrasound To Improve the Diagnostic Accuracy of Surgical Exploration

Intraoperative ultrasonography has been used to identify a variety of intracranial abnormalities, including ventricular enlargement, intra- and extra-axial tumors, and arteriovenous malformations,[6,7,10] as well as to guide needle biopsy of deep intracranial lesions[4,6,7,10,12] and stereotactic placement of electrodes,[4] radioactive implants,[13] and ventricular shunts in infants.[9] Since 1985, we have used this technique to improve the diagnostic accuracy of burr-hole exploration and subsequent craniotomy in severely head-injured patients with clinical signs of brain stem compression.

Although complete, bilateral burr-hole exploration can rapidly and accurately identify traumatic extra-axial hematomas and speed their surgical evacuation, it may not detect intracerebral hematomas (see Chapter 7).[3] Because intracranial blood is highly echogenic, however, real-time, high-resolution ultrasonography can detect these lesions with exquisite sensitivity.[8] In an experimental study, intracerebral hematomas as small as 2 cc were readily detected as well-circumscribed, homogenous, brightly echogenic lesions surrounded by normal hypoechoic brain.[8]

From *Traumatic Transtentorial Herniation and Its Management* by Brian T. Andrews, MD and Lawrence H. Pitts, MD © 1991, Futura Publishing Co., Inc., Mount Kisco, NY.

In this chapter, we describe the use of high-resolution, real-time ultrasonography during surgical exploration and summarize our experience with these techniques in a series of 31 head-injured patients with clinical signs of brain stem compression.

Ultrasound Method

In the operating room, the epidural and subdural spaces are examined through bilateral temporal, frontal, and parietal burr-holes. If a significant epidural or subdural hematoma is encountered, the exposure is immediately converted to a large craniotomy, and the hematoma is evacuated. If no extra-axial mass lesion is encountered but the brain appears to be tense or herniating out of the dural opening or if there is visual evidence of cortical contusions, intraoperative ultrasonography may be performed to further evaluate the brain parenchyma. After evacuation of an epidural or subdural hematoma, ultrasonography may be performed through the craniotomy defect to identify intracerebral hematomas and to evaluate persistent brain swelling.

We use a Diasonics® (Model S2, Milpitas, CA) real-time ultrasound sector scanner and a high-resolution probe. A 7.5-MHz probe can identify lesions less than 3 cm from the cortical surface, and a 5-MHz probe can identify lesions 3–7 cm deep. More recently, we have used a 3.5-MHz probe, which can penetrate to a depth of 10–15 cm. The tip of the probe is placed into one finger of a sterile latex glove, and the probe and cable are sterilely draped using an arthroscope drape (Xomed Inc. Jacksonville, FL).

Ultrasonography is performed by the neurosurgeon through the dura or on the cortical surface through each burr-hole or the craniotomy site (Fig. 9-1) to a depth that shows the midline structures, including the falx (Fig. 9-2). In children and smaller adults, the 3.5-MHz probe can accurately evaluate both hemispheres of the brain through a unilateral set of burr-holes or a craniotomy[2] (Fig. 9-3). Intra-axial lesions that appear to be echodense are interpreted as intracerebral hematomas if they are confluent (Fig. 9-4) and as cerebral contusions if they are not.[1,5] The decision to remove or not to remove a mass lesion identified by ultrasonography depends upon its size, location, and the degree of mass effect on surrounding brain.[1,11]

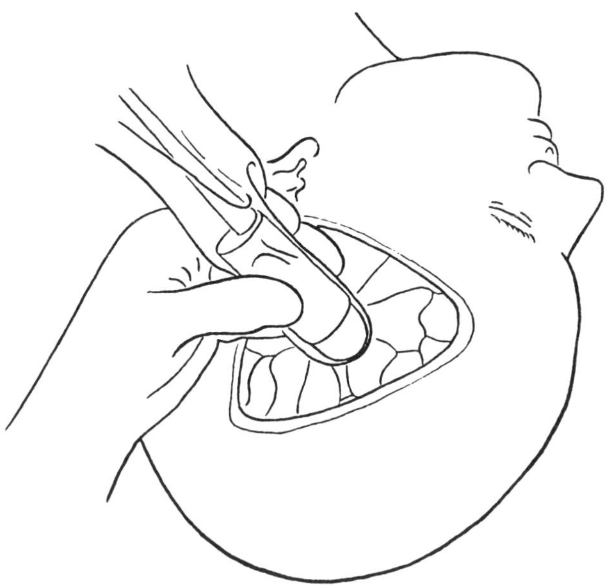

Figure 9-1. Ultrasound probe draped in sterile fashion and positioned over the brain surface to evaluate the brain parenchyma for the presence of intracerebral hematomas.

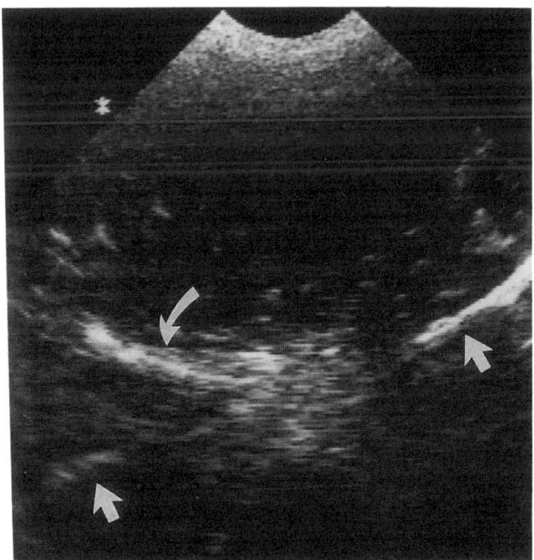

Figure 9-2. Intraoperative ultrasound image of normal brain parenchyma from the surface of the frontal cortex showing the midline falx *(arrows)* and the adjacent choroid plexus *(curved arrow)*.

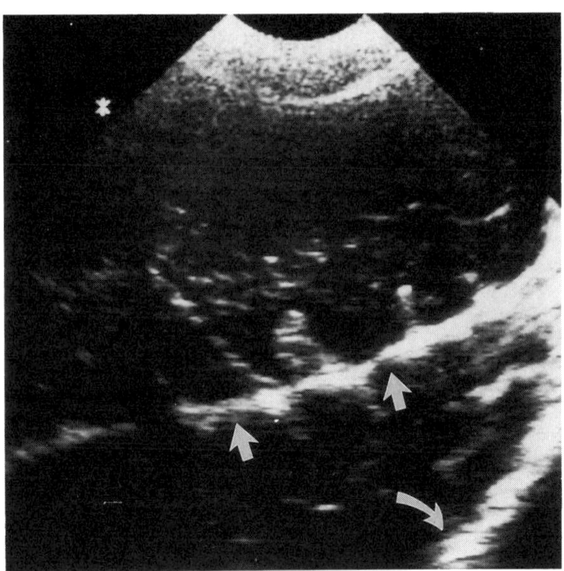

Figure 9-3. Intraoperative ultrasound image from a frontal burr-hole showing the falx cerebrum *(straight arrows)*, the entire width of the brain, and the contralateral convexity *(curved arrow)*. Intraoperative ultrasonography allows evaluation of the contralateral epidural and subdural spaces through a unilateral set of burr-holes or a craniotomy.

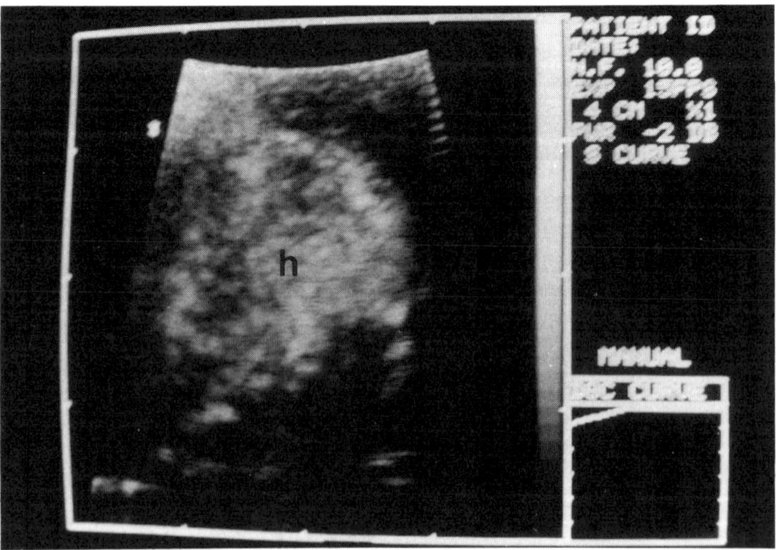

Figure 9-4. Intraoperative ultrasound image showing an intracerebral hemorrhage (h) as an area of homogenously increased echogenicity.

Clinical Application

Between January 1, 1984, and December 31, 1988, 20 patients, including 17 previously reported,[1] were evaluated with bilateral and 11 with unilateral intraoperative ultrasonography. All patients had severe head injuries and clinical signs of transtentorial herniation. Significant extra-axial mass lesions were detected by burr-hole exploration and evacuated through a craniotomy in 22 (71%) of the 31 patients. Twenty-one patients had subdural hematomas, which were bilateral in four cases and ipsilateral to an epidural hematoma in three. One patient had an isolated epidural hematoma. Surgical exploration revealed obvious brain contusions in four patients.

Bilateral ultrasonography of each hemisphere separately showed no intracerebral mass in 15 (75%) of 20 patients. In one patient who had a negative burr-hole exploration, a small intraparenchymal hematoma was identified in the region of the basal ganglia of the dominant hemisphere but was not evacuated. Among four patients who underwent a craniotomy to evacuate a hematoma, the ultrasound examination showed extensive contusions of the temporal lobe. This finding contributed to the decision to perform a partial temporal lobectomy in two. In each case, some superficial contusion was visible through the craniotomy, but its extent was best demonstrated by ultrasonography.

Ultrasonography of the entire brain through a unilateral exposure confirmed the absence of significant intracerebral mass lesions in nine of 11 patients. In one patient, ultrasonography demonstrated diffuse bilateral cerebral contusions and intraventricular hemorrhage. In another patient, who had a craniotomy to evacuate a subdural hematoma, the examination revealed a contralateral subdural hematoma, which was immediately evacuated through a second craniotomy.

The findings of intraoperative ultrasonography were confirmed by CT scanning in 18 patients and by autopsy in 10 who died during or soon after surgery. In three patients (10%), CT scans showed small but significant lesions not identified by ultrasound examination. In two of the patients, ultrasound missed a mass lesion at the ipsilateral frontal pole after evacuation of a subdural hematoma identified by burr-hole exploration. One had a residual subdural hematoma that was evacuated immediately; the other had a small intraparenchymal hemorrhage that subsequently enlarged and was evacuated 36 hours later. These two lesions were anterior to the usual frontal burr-hole site, which is just anterior to the coronal suture. To improve the ultrasonographic demonstration of the anterior frontal lobe, we now rongeur the inner table at the frontal burr-hole. The third patient had a significant temporal lobe hematoma that was evacuated through a subsequent craniotomy. Because the CT scan was obtained some hours after the burr-hole exploration and ultrasound examination proved negative, the temporal lesion was considered by the operating neurosurgeons to be a delayed rather than a missed hematoma.

Intraoperative ultrasound imaging accurately identified or ruled out intracerebral mass lesions in 88% of cases. Among patients with negative burr-holes, the results of ultrasonography were confirmed by CT immediately after surgery in each case. Ultrasonography also provided information on the size and location of hemorrhagic contusions that helped to decide whether or not to resect the damaged brain. The results of this study support our recommendation to perform diagnostic burr-hole exploration before CT scanning in patients with clinical evidence of brain stem compression after head injury. Although the incidence of intracerebral hematomas immediately after trauma is low,[1,3] such lesions can usually be identified by intraoperative ultrasonography during burr-hole exploration and evacuated expediently.

References

1. Andrews B, Bederson JB, Pitts LH: Use of intraoperative ultrasonography to improve the diagnostic accuracy of exploratory burr holes in patients with traumatic tentorial herniation. Neurosurgery 24:345-347, 1989.
2. Andrews BT, Mampalam TJ, Omsberg E, Pitts LH: Intraoperative ultrasound imaging of the entire brain through unilateral exploratory burr holes after severe head injury. Surg Neurol 33:1990. In press.
3. Andrews BT, Pitts LH, Lovely MP, et al.: Is computed tomographic scanning necessary in patients with tentorial herniation? Results of immediate surgical exploration without computerized tomography in 100 patients. Neurosurgery 19:408-414, 1986.
4. Berger MS: Ultrasound-guided stereotaxic biopsy using a new apparatus. J Neurosurg 65:550-554, 1986.

5. Brown FD, Rachlin JR, Rubin JM, et al.: Ultrasound-guided periventricular stereotaxis. Neurosurgery 15:162-164, 1984.
6. Chandler WF, Knake JE, McGillicuddy JE, et al.: Intraoperative use of real-time ultrasonography in neurosurgery. J Neurosurg 57:157-163, 1982.
7. Dohrmann GJ, Rubin JM: Use of ultrasound in neurosurgical operations: a preliminary report. Surg Neurol 16:362-366, 1981.
8. Enzmann DR, Britt RH, Lyons B, et al.: Experimental study of high-resolution ultrasound imaging of hemorrhage, bone fragment, and foreign bodies in head trauma. J Neurosurg 54:304-309, 1981.
9. Shkolnik A, McLone DG: Intraoperative real-time ultrasonic guidance of ventricular shunt placement in infants. Radiology 141:515-517, 1981.
10. Sjolander U, Lindgren PG, Hugosson R: Ultrasound sector scanning for the localization and biopsy of intracerebral lesions. J Neurosurg 58:7-10, 1983.
11. Soloniuk D, Pitts LH, Lovely M, et al. Traumatic intracerebral hematomas: timing of appearance and indications for operative removal. J Trauma 26:787-793, 1986.
12. Tsutsumi Y, Andoh Y, Inoue N: Ultrasound-guided biopsy for deep-seated brain tumors. J Neurosurg 57:164-167, 1982.
13. Tsutsumi Y, Andoh Y, Matsutani M, et al.: New technique for removable implantation of radionuclides in central nervous system neoplasm by ultrasonic guidance. Surg Neurol 23:520-524, 1985.

CHAPTER 10

Burr-Hole Exploration in Children

Our studies of emergency burr-hole exploration in head-injured patients with clinical signs of brain stem compression have shown that the incidence of extra-axial mass lesions is age-related (see Chapter 7). Among 100 such patients, only 36% of those younger than 30 years of age had positive surgical results, compared with 60% of those 30 to 59 years of age and 75% of those 60 years and older.[3] Low-speed injuries, such as falls or vehicle-pedestrian accidents, were the most common mechanism of injury in patients with mass lesions.[4] Nevertheless, in our population, more than 50% of children with clinical signs of traumatic transtentorial herniation have significant extra-axial hematomas, typically after a low-speed injury. In this chapter, we describe the clinical and operative findings in a consecutive series of head-injured children with clinical signs of brain stem compression who underwent emergency burr-hole exploration between January 1, 1981, and December 31, 1986.[3]

Methods

The children were taken to the emergency room, evaluated, and resuscitated as described in Chapters 3 and 4. In all cases, the trauma team included an attending pediatrician experienced in trauma care. The surgical exploration differed from that in adults only in that particular attention was paid to minimizing operative blood loss,

From *Traumatic Transtentorial Herniation and Its Management* by Brian T. Andrews, MD and Lawrence H. Pitts, MD © 1991, Futura Publishing Co., Inc., Mount Kisco, NY.

and the hematocrit and hemodynamic status were carefully monitored and supported with crystalloid solutions, blood transfusions, and pressor agents (e.g., dopamine), if necessary. Arterial carbon dioxide tension was maintained at 20–25 mm Hg by hyperventilation until the surgical findings were known. Intracranial pressure monitoring was initiated as soon as possible in all patients. If it was less than 20 mm Hg initially, hyperventilation was decreased as tolerated to maintain normal intracranial pressure.

Burr-hole exploration was performed as described in Chapter 7, including the use of intraoperative ultrasonography to identify intraparenchymal hematomas and contusions.[1] Since 1986 we have used a 3.5-MHz ultrasound probe, which allows greater depth of penetration and, in children, because of the smaller size of the calvarium, can show both hemispheres of the brain and the contralateral convexity through unilateral frontal, temporal, and parietal burr-holes (see Chapter 9).

Late outcome was determined using the Glasgow Outcome Scale.[14] Children were considered vegetative if they remained unresponsive to the environment, severely disabled if they were conscious but dependent, moderately disabled if they had not returned to their previous level of schooling or verbal and motor function, and as having made a good recovery if they returned to their previous functional level with little or no impairment. An autopsy was performed on all children who died.

Summary of Cases

Clinical Findings

There were 10 boys and seven girls, 11 months to 17 years of age (mean 7.3 years). Six patients were less than 3 years of age, six were 3 to 9, four were 10 to 15, and one was 17. Nine children were injured in vehicle-pedestrian accidents, five in falls, and three as motor vehicle occupants. Only one child had a witnessed lucid interval before arrival in the emergency room. The physical findings at admission are shown in Table 10-1. Four of the five patients with major internal injuries underwent a thoracotomy in the emergency room.

Table 10-1 Physical Findings in 17 Patients at Admission

Finding	*No. of patients*
Cardiac arrest	2
Hypotension	
(systolic blood pressure < 90 mm Hg)	3
Major thoracic or abdominal injury	5
Lateralizing neurological findings	
Single dilated pupil	10 (59%)
Hemiparesis or hemiplegia	5
Nonlateralizing neurological findings	
Bilaterally dilated pupils	7 (41%)
Bilateral localizing to pain	1
Bilateral flexor-extensor posturing	2
Bilateral flaccidity	9 (53%)
Glasgow coma score*	
Score of 3	10 (59%)

*Median score, 3; range, 3–10.

Surgical Findings

The surgical findings are shown in Table 10-2. Burr-hole exploration identified an extra-axial mass lesion in nine (53%) of 17 patients. Each of these patients had a subdural hematoma, which was immediately evacuated; in one, the hematoma was small and may not have caused the signs of brain stem compression seen at admission. In one child without an extra-axial lesion, a small, deep-seated intraparenchymal hemorrhage in the dominant hemisphere was diagnosed by intraoperative ultrasonography but was not removed because of its small size and location. In another child, a depressed skull fracture was identified and reduced. Thus, intracranial abnormalities were identified during surgical exploration in 11 of 17 patients (65%).

Table 10-2 Surgical Findings in 17 Patients

Finding	*No. of patients*
Positive exploration	11 (65%)
Extra-axial hematoma	9
Intraparenchymal hematoma	1
Depressed skull fracture	1
Negative exploration	6

The surgical findings appeared to be independent of age, lateralizing neurological findings (including anisocoria), and the mechanism of trauma, but correlated strongly with systemic hypotension or cardiac arrest at admission. Only one (16.6%) of six patients with abnormally low blood pressure had an intracranial hematoma, compared with eight (73%) of 11 patients whose blood pressure was normal (chi-square = 7.46, $p < 0.01$).

CT scans, obtained immediately after the operation in 12 children, confirmed the intraoperative findings in each case. No child had an extra-axial or intraparenchymal hematoma that was not detected during surgical exploration. Among the five survivors who had positive burr-hole explorations, the clinical signs of brain stem compression diminished or resolved in the early postoperative period. In no case did autopsy reveal an intracranial mass not diagnosed by burr-hole exploration.

Outcome

The outcome in each patient is summarized in Table 10-3. Nine children (53%) survived, and eight (47%) died. Five of the children who died had major thoracic or abdominal injury and cardiac arrest or systemic hypotension at admission. The survival rate was slightly better among children in whom a subdural hematoma was evacuated than in those with negative surgical findings (56% vs. 50%).

After a mean follow-up period of 15.2 months (range, 6 to 72 months), seven (78%) of the nine patients that survived had made a good recovery, and two were moderately disabled. No child was severely disabled or vegetative. Subdural hematomas were evacuated in four of the patients who had a good outcome and in one who

Table 10-3 Outcome in 17 Patients

Outcome	*No. of patients*
Good recovery	7 (41%)
Moderately disabled	2 (12%)
Severely disabled	0
Vegetative	0
Dead	8 (47%)
Within 6 hours of operation	2 (12%)
Within 7 days of operation	6 (35%)

was moderately disabled. The only patient with hypotension at admission who survived had a good outcome. Age did not appear to correlate with the mortality rate or with functional outcome.

Discussion

The higher incidence of mass lesions in children in this study than in similarly injured young adults in our earlier study (53% vs. 36%)[3] may relate to a variety of physiological, anatomical, or epidemiological differences. The relatively greater cranial volume and weaker cervical musculature in children may increase the risk of head injury caused by less forceful trauma, as in the so-called shaken-baby syndrome.[9,11,13] Children also have relatively larger venous sinuses, which may render them more susceptible to the development of intracranial mass lesions after trauma.

The mechanism of trauma may also affect the incidence of mass lesions after head injury. Young adults are most frequently injured as occupants in motor vehicle accidents.[3,6,7] Bowers and Marshall[6] reported that extra-axial hematomas are rare in patients with severe head injury caused by motor vehicle accidents. We have found that positive burr-hole explorations are much more common after low-speed injuries, such as falls and vehicle-pedestrian accidents, than after high-speed injuries sustained in motor vehicle accidents, regardless of the age of the patient.[3] Jellinger[13] has also reported that among children, acute subdural hematomas most often result from mechanisms such as falls or battered-child syndrome. All but three of our pediatric patients were injured in falls or vehicle-pedestrian accidents, and nine (53%) had extra-axial hematomas. In an earlier series from our institution, 46% of severely head-injured children had an intracranial hematoma, and 95% had suffered low-speed trauma.[5]

Other studies of children with severe head injury, however, have shown that diffuse cerebral swelling is more common than intracranial mass lesions. In the series of Bruce et al.,[7] only 12 (23%) of 53 children had intracranial hematomas; but 38 (72%) were injured in motor vehicle accidents, and a minority suffered low-speed trauma. The higher incidence of extra-axial mass lesions in severely head-injured children in our study may simply indicate that falls, vehicle-pedestrian accidents, and other types of low-speed trauma are a much more common cause of severe head injury in San Francisco than are motor vehicle accidents.[3,5] Clearly, the incidence of mass lesions varies from city to city, depending upon the mechanisms of head injury common to each region.

Burr-hole exploration before CT scanning has been criticized because of the potential for missing intracerebral hemorrhages. These lesions, however, are rare immediately after trauma, in children as well as adults.[5,13,18] Berger et al.[5] reported that only two (5%) of 38 children with severe head injury had isolated intracerebral hemorrhages; three others had both intracerebral and extra-axial hematomas. In the current series, only one child (6%) had an intracerebral hematoma, which was deep within the dominant hemisphere and did not require evacuation. This lesion was identified by intraoperative real-time ultrasonography at the time of burr-hole exploration. Use of this technique obviates the need for preoperative CT scanning to identify parenchymal lesions that might potentially be missed at the time of surgery (see Chapter 9). The relatively smaller cranial vault in children allows acceptable imaging of both cerebral hemispheres and convexities with a 3.5-MHz ultrasound probe through unilateral frontal, temporal, and parietal burr-holes and may allow surgical exploration to be limited to one hemisphere if the contralateral convexity can be adequately demonstrated and is free of mass lesions.

Cardiac arrest or systemic hypotension at admission was associated with a low incidence of intracranial hematomas and was the only clinical factor that correlated with the surgical findings. In patients with abnormally low blood pressure, clinical signs of brain stem dysfunction probably indicate primary ischemia, rather than compression, of the brain stem; but when the systolic blood pressure remains above 60 mm Hg, signs of tentorial herniation or brain stem compression reliably reflect the presence of an intracranial mass lesion (see Chapter 5). Severe hypotension or cardiac arrest may also limit bleeding into the subdural or epidural spaces and thereby reduce the likelihood that a significant extra-axial hematoma would develop before surgical exploration.[8] The results of the present study further support these findings: burr-hole exploration demonstrated an extra-axial mass lesion in only one (16.6%) of six children who had severe hypotension or initial cardiac arrest, but in eight (73%) of 11 of those who did not.

The outcome among children in this series is remarkable for the lower mortality rate than among similarly injured adults and the high level of neurological recovery among the survivors. In recent series of adults with signs of transtentorial herniation after severe head injury, the mortality rate has usually been greater than 70%.[3,10,12,15,17] In contrast, the mortality rate in this series was 47%, and five of the eight children who died had multiple, severe systemic injuries and severe hypotension or cardiac arrest at admission; these factors are associated with a sharply increased mortality rate after severe head injury.[16] In the series of Berger et al.,[5] 52% of severely head-injured children had a good outcome or were moderately disabled. The results in the current series are even more remarkable in that all of the children had clinical signs of brain stem compression, and the mean initial Glasgow coma score was lower than in the series of Berger et al.[5] In the series of Bruce et al.,[7] in which intracranial mass lesions were less common than diffuse cerebral swelling (23% vs. 34%), 90% of children had a good outcome or were moderately disabled. Signs of brain stem compression, systemic injuries, and cardiovascular instability were less common in their series than in ours.

Seven of the nine survivors in the current series had a good outcome, and none were severely disabled or vegetative. In contrast, 10%–25% of similarly injured adults who survive have a nonfunctional outcome.[3,12,15,17] Although Berger et al. reported that severely head-injured children under 5 years of age more frequently achieve an independent outcome (good recovery or moderate disability) than older children,[5] we found no such difference in our study.

Conclusion

In San Francisco, more than 50% of children with clinical signs of transtentorial herniation or brain stem dysfunction after trauma have extra-axial hematomas; among those without severe hypotension or initial cardiac arrest, the incidence exceeds 70%. The high incidence of mass lesions may be related to the predominance of low-speed injuries, such as falls and vehicle-pedestrian accidents, among children in our metropolitan area, and the relatively young age of the children in this series. Patients such as ours may be reasonably managed by emergency burr-hole exploration, complemented by intraoperative ultrasonography, to detect and evacuate extra-axial and intra-axial hematomas as rapidly as possible. This approach avoids the delay inherent in performing a CT scan, but may submit the patient to "unnecessary surgery" if the burr-holes are negative.

In metropolitan or rural areas where high-speed motor vehicle accidents are the most common cause of head injuries in children, the incidence of intracranial mass lesions may be lower, even among children with clinical signs of brain stem dysfunction. In such patients, it is eminently reasonable to perform an emergency CT scan rather than burr-hole exploration. Among children with initial systemic hypotension or cardiac arrest, clinical signs of brain stem dysfunction do not reliably predict an intracranial mass lesion, and an initial CT scan should be obtained, if possible, before surgical intervention.

References

1. Andrews BT, Bederson J, Pitts LH: The use of intraoperative ultrasound to improve the diagnostic accuracy of exploratory burr holes in traumatic tentorial herniation. Neurosurgery 24: 345-347, 1989.
2. Andrews BT, Levy ML, Pitts LH: Implications of systemic hypotension for the neurological examination in patients with severe head injury. Surg Neurol 28:419-422, 1987.
3. Andrews BT, Pitts LH, Lovely MP, et al.: Is computed tomographic scanning necessary in patients with tentorial herniation? Results of immediate surgical exploration without computerized tomography in 100 patients. Neurosurgery 19:408-414, 1986.
4. Andrews BT, Ross AM, Pitts LH: Surgical exploration before computed tomography scanning in children with traumatic tentorial herniation. Surg Neurol 32:434-438, 1989.
5. Berger MS, Pitts LH, Lovely M, et al.: Outcome from severe head injury in children and adolescents. J Neurosurg 62:194-199, 1985.
6. Bowers SA, Marshall LF: Outcome in 200 consecutive cases of severe head injury treated in San Diego County: a prospective analysis. Neurosurgery 6:237-242, 1980.
7. Bruce DA, Schut L, Bruno LA, et al.: Outcome following severe head injuries in children. J Neurosurg 48:679-688, 1978.

8. Bucci MN, Phillips TW, McGillicuddy JE: Delayed epidural hemorrhage in hypotensive multiple trauma patients. Neurosurgery 19:65-68, 1986.
9. Duhaime AC, Gennarelli TA, Thibault LE, et al.: The shaken baby syndrome. A clinical, pathological, and biomechanical study. J Neurosurg 66:409-415, 1987.
10. Gutterman P, Shenken HA: Prognostic features in recovery from traumatic decerebration. J Neurosurg 32:330-335, 1979.
11. Hadley MN, Sonntag VKH, Rekate HL, et al.: The infant whiplash-shake syndrome: A clinical and pathological study. Neurosurgery 24:536-540, 1989.
12. Hoff JT, Spetzler R, Winestock D: Head injury and early signs of tentorial herniation—a management dilemma. West J Med 128: 112-116, 1978.
13. Jellinger K: The neuropathology of pediatric head injuries. In Shapiro K (ed): Pediatric Head Trauma. Mount Kisco, NY: Futura Publishing Co. 1983, pp 143-194.
14. Jennett B, Bond M: Assessment of outcome after severe brain damage: a practical scale. Lancet 1:480-484, 1975.
15. Mahoney BD, Rockswold GL, Ruiz E, et al.: Emergency twist-drill trephination. Neurosurgery 8:551-554, 1981.
16. Newfield P, Pitts LH, Kaktis J: Influence of shock on survival after head trauma. Neurosurgery 6:596, 1980.
17. Seelig JM, Greenberg RP, Becker DP, et al.: Reversible brain stem dysfunction following acute traumatic subdural hematoma—a clinical and electrophysiological study. J Neurosurg 55:550-554, 1986
18. Soloniuk D, Pitts LH, Lovely M, et al.: Traumatic intracerebral hematomas: timing of appearance and indications for operative removal. J Trauma 29:787-793, 1986.

CHAPTER 11

Intensive Care Management

After initial diagnostic and therapeutic measures have been completed, including evacuation of intracranial hematomas if present, placement of an intracranial pressure (ICP) monitor, and the acute management of other systemic injuries, the patient is taken to the intensive care unit (ICU). The goals of intensive care for patients with transtentorial herniation are the same as for any patient with a severe head injury. These include frequent assessments to identify neurological deterioration; continuous monitoring of ICP and treatment to control ICP elevation; continuous monitoring and management of arterial blood pressure to prevent hypotension or excessive hypertension and to maintain adequate cerebral perfusion pressure (CPP); continued endotracheal intubation and controlled ventilation to assure an adequate airway and tissue oxygenation and, if necessary, to control ICP elevation by hyperventilation; and monitoring of nutritional and infectious disease status to allow early institution of nutritional support and prompt treatment of infections. Additional intensive care measures for various systemic or orthopedic injuries are tailored to specific needs.

Neurological Assessment

Throughout the patient's stay in the ICU, the neurological status is assessed hourly to identify neurological deterioration. Delayed complications of head injury include intracerebral hematomas, enlarged hemorrhagic contusions with cerebral edema, and increased

From *Traumatic Transtentorial Herniation and Its Management* by Brian T. Andrews, MD and Lawrence H. Pitts, MD © 1991, Futura Publishing Co., Inc., Mount Kisco, NY.

ICP. The neurological assessment is usually performed hourly by the ICU nursing staff, verified periodically by the neurosurgeon or neurosurgical resident, and recorded on a flow sheet (Fig. 11-1). The data recorded include the Glasgow coma score (eye opening, verbal, and motor responses),[44] pupillary function, limb strength, and the highest ICP during the previous hour.[33]

Neurological deterioration should be verified by the neurosurgeon and evaluated in light of the patient's clinical course and treatment. It is especially important to consider factors that could affect the neurological status, including such drugs as anticonvulsants, morphine, or barbiturates and conditions such as systemic hypotension, hypoxia, or hyperthermia. If none of these factors are present, and if the neurological deterioration is progressive and substantial, computerized tomography (CT) may be necessary to identify or rule out a hematoma or other delayed intracranial complications.[1]

Monitoring of Intracranial Pressure

We continuously monitor ICP in all severely head-injured patients for a minimum of 48 hours after injury or until the ICP remains below 15 mm Hg without treatment for at least 24 hours. Continuous monitoring has several advantages. First, it identifies elevated ICP, which can produce a decrease in CPP, calculated as MAP-ICP, where MAP is the mean arterial pressure. Treatment of ICP greater than 20 mm Hg has been widely recommended[4,8,16,23,33,42,47] to maintain CPP above approximately 60 mm Hg.

Second, ICP monitoring can provide an early warning of delayed complication of head injury. Progressive elevation in ICP may indicate a developing intracerebral hematoma or an enlarging hemorrhagic contusion with cerebral edema.[1,33,42] This is important because mass lesions may cause little change in the results of neurological examination, particularly in deeply comatose patients.

Third, ICP monitoring data are useful for predicting the prognosis for recovery and, in some patients with fatal head injury, for determi-

Figure 11-1. (Facing page) Flow sheet used to record hourly neurological observations in the intensive care unit allows graphic identification of neurological deterioration, including changes in pupillary function, Glasgow coma score, and limb movement.

Neuro Flowsheet

Glasgow Coma Scale

Pupil Scale (m.m.)	1	2	3	4	5	6	7	8
	•	●	●	●	●	●	●	●

		Date																								
		Time	07	08	09	10	11	12	13	14	15	16	17	18	19	20	21	22	23	24	01	02	03	04	05	06
PUPILS	right	Size																								
		Reaction																								
	left	Size																								
		Reaction																								
COMA SCALE	Eyes Open	4 Spontaneously																								
		3 To speech																								
		2 To pain																								
		1 To none																								
	Best Motor Response	6 Obey commands																								
		5 Localize pain																								
		4 Flexion withdrawl																								
		3 Flexion normal																								
		2 Extension																								
		1 None																								
	Best Response to Auditory/ Visual Stimulus	**ADULT**																								
		5 Orientation																								
		4 Confused																								
		3 Inappropriate words																								
		2 Incomprehensible words																								
		1 None																								
		T= Endotracheal Tube or Tracheostomy																								
		L= Language Barrier																								
	COMA SCALE TOTALS																									
LIMB MOVEMENT			R/L	R/L	R/L	R/L	R/L	R/L	R/L	R/L	R/L	R/L	R/L	R/L	R/L	R/L	R/L	R/L	R/L	R/L	R/L	R/L	R/L	R/L	R/L	R/L
	ARMS	Voluntary motor (0-5)																								
		Flexion withdrawl																								
		Flexion Abnormal																								
		Extension																								
		No Response																								
	LEGS	Voluntary motor (0-5)																								
		Flexion																								
		Extension																								
		No Response																								
		MAP																								
		ICP																								

++ = brisk
+ = sluggish
- = no reaction
C = eye closed by swelling

Eyes closed by swelling = C

+ = Present
- = Absent
NT = Not Tested
0 = No Movement
1 = Trace Movement
2 = Movement, but not against gravity
3 = Movement against gravity, but not against resistance
4 = Movement against gravity and some resistance
5 = Full Power

Children's Hospital of San Francisco KD 5/89

Figure 11–1.

ning brain death (see Chapter 13). If the ICP is equal to or greater than the MAP, there is no cerebral perfusion and blood flow to the brain stops. When it is appropriate to declare brain death, ICP data may supplant other measures of cerebral perfusion, such as radionuclide brain scans, transcranial Doppler studies, or cerebral arteriography.

Placement of the ICP Monitor

During burr-hole exploration, we routinely place a catheter in the subdural space, which is brought out through the skin for continuous ICP monitoring[3] (Fig. 11-2). Subdural catheter systems have

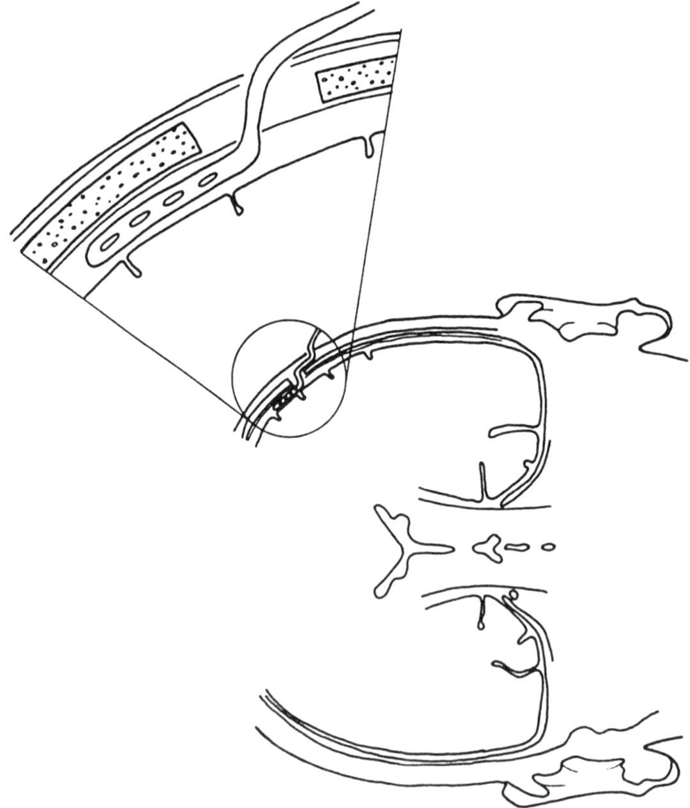

Figure 11-2. Diagram showing a subdural intracranial pressure monitor in place after burr-hole exploration or craniotomy. The catheter is filled with normal saline solution and connected to a transducer calibrated in mm Hg.

proven to be accurate and reliable and may be more easily placed than intraventricular catheters,[29] especially if the cerebral ventricles are small. However, an intraventricular catheter may be useful because it allows drainage of cerebrospinal fluid (CSF) as a method of lowering ICP.[8,27] Some neurosurgeons continue to use a subarachnoid bolt,[50] although there is a tendency for such systems to become obstructed by brain tissue and lose accuracy,[29] particularly if ICP is markedly elevated. Recently, fiber-optic catheter systems have been introduced[31] that are also easily placed and can provide accurate long-term monitoring of ICP.

Management of Elevated Intracranial Pressure

A key goal of the management of severely head-injured patients, with or without clinical signs of transtentorial herniation, is to reduce elevated ICP and maintain an adequate CPP. Normal CPP is approximately 80–90 mm Hg. In normal brain, cerebral autoregulation fails and cerebral blood flow (CBF) begins to fall when CPP is less than 50 mm Hg. In injured regions of the brain, where focal tissue pressure may be higher than the mean ICP, a CPP of 50 mm Hg may be too low for optimal perfusion. Therefore, CPP should be maintained above 60 mm Hg to assure adequate cerebral perfusion,[8,47] especially in the injured brain. Given the need for an adequate CPP, preventing increased ICP and maintaining MAP are critical. The most common and effective methods for treating elevated ICP are controlled hyperventilation and intravenous infusion of mannitol or furosemide (Table 11-1).

Table 11-1 Management of Elevated Intracranial Pressure
Controlled hyperventilation (Pa_{CO_2} approximately 25 mm Hg)
Mannitol (0.25–0.5 g/kg, given as an intravenous bolus)
Sedation for restlessness
Head of the bed elevated 20°
Furosemide
Barbiturates

Hyperventilation

Hyperventilation decreases arterial carbon dioxide tension (Pa_{CO_2}) and increases the pH of blood and extracellular fluids and thus induces a respiratory alkalosis. Because increased serum pH is a primary and potent cause for cerebral arteriolar vasodilatation, respiratory alkalosis causes cerebral vasoconstriction.[8,17,18,25,33] Vasoconstriction decreases the cerebral blood volume, and thus the volume of the brain, immediately lowering the ICP. Hyperventilation progressively increases cerebral vasoconstriction until $Paco_2$ declines to approximately 20 mm Hg; additional hyperventilation to decrease $Paco_2$ below this level may not result in further vasoconstriction[32,37] and therefore, to avoid metabolic complications from excessive serum alkalosis, is seldom employed. A $Paco_2$ below 20 mm Hg may reduce CBF below the level needed to maintain normal metabolism.[16] Vasoconstriction induced by hyperventilation is more pronounced in areas of the brain with intact autoregulation. Paul et al.[32] have shown that patients with a diffuse brain injury and loss of cerebral autoregulation are less responsive to hyperventilation than those with more focal abnormalities or injury primarily to the brain stem.

The duration of the effect of hyperventilation has recently been investigated experimentally by Muizelaar et al.[25] Continuous hyperventilation to maintain a $Paco_2$ of 25 mm Hg resulted in a steady loss of pial arteriolar vasoconstriction. After 20 hours, vessel diameters were slightly above baseline values; subsequent return to normocapnia resulted in vasodilatation and an increase in cerebral blood volume. During the same period, arterial and CSF pH had also normalized. Similar pH and blood volume findings have been found during prolonged hyperventilation in humans.[7,18] These results suggest that after 20 to 24 hours, continuous hyperventilation may lose its effect, and later attempts to normalize $Paco_2$ may cause vasodilatation and increased ICP. We therefore recommend that hyperventilation be used only to treat acute elevations in ICP[33] and not to prevent increases in ICP, as has been suggested.[4,42] For subsequent control of ICP, we attempt to normalize the $Paco_2$ as much as tolerated to maintain arteriolar CO_2 responsiveness and allow us to use hyperventilation again if necessary.

Severely head-injured patients commonly suffer from hypoxia and hypoventilation as a result of lung or chest injuries or CNS-induced hypoventilation. Such insults may lead to cerebral vasodilatation, adding to other causes of increased ICP. Administering oxygen to maintain the Pao_2 above 100 mm Hg may reverse these detrimental pulmonary conditions. In addition, the respiratory alkalosis induced by hyperventilation tends to reduce intracerebral acidosis, which may aid brain recovery. Direct injuries to the chest that could inhibit adequate ventilation must be appropriately managed. Penetrating chest trauma that results in pneumothorax or hemothorax requires placement of a chest tube and thoracotomy. Blunt chest trauma, such as rib fractures, a flail segment of the chest, or pulmonary contusions, may lead to pulmonary insufficiency and usually necessitates positive-pressure ventilation.

Mannitol

In addition to hyperventilation as a means of lowering ICP, we routinely administer intravenous mannitol, 0.25–0.5 g/kg, as often as every 4–6 hours. Mannitol, a 6-carbon sugar similar to glucose, is not metabolized and remains primarily in the intravascular and extracellular spaces.[16] Wise and Chater[51] were the first to show that CSF pressure and brain mass decrease after intravenous infusion of mannitol. Infusion of hypertonic mannitol into the intravascular space causes osmotic dehydration of the brain, which reduces the volume of extracellular free water.[41] Mannitol infusion has several additional effects: it immediately increases the circulating blood volume, which increases systemic arterial blood pressure,[51] and causes hemodilution, which reduces blood viscosity.[5,26] In addition, red blood cell deformability is increased and blood viscosity is decreased; neither of these effects is related to hemodilution.[5] Mannitol also improves intracranial compliance out of proportion to its effect in reducing ICP.[19]

Muizelaar et al.[26] have shown experimentally that cerebral vasoconstriction occurs in direct response to the decrease in blood viscosity that follows mannitol infusion. They postulate that decreased blood viscosity leads to improved red cell oxygen transport, which, when autoregulation is intact, results in vasoconstriction.[24,26] Rosner et al.[41] have shown that ICP responds better to mannitol in patients with a low initial CPP than in those with a high CPP. They suggest that the effect of mannitol on systemic arterial blood pressure increases CPP and allows direct cerebral vasoconstriction. Thus, mannitol infusion may result in cerebral vasoconstriction and lower ICP through several mechanisms, in addition to its osmotic effects on the brain.

Repeated administration of mannitol usually results in a hyperosmolar state, i.e., serum osmolality and dehydration. Hyperosmolar agents should not be used when osmolality rises above 340 mM, which can cause neural cell dysfunction and cardiopulmonary and renal complications.[33] Excessive fluid loss should also be avoided, and lost fluid should be replaced to avoid excessive dehydration and decreased cardiac output. Clifton[8] recommends using a Swan-Ganz catheter to monitor the pulmonary wedge pressure and measure cardiac output; the wedge pressure should be maintained above 5 mm Hg. Others recommend that central venous pressure be monitored to guide the administration of fluids to maintain a central venous pressure of 2–5 mm Hg.[45]

Furosemide

Furosemide has long been used to reduce intracerebral free water and brain edema.[8,9,33,42,43] It appears to act, in part, through diuresis, which increases intravascular oncotic pressure and forces extracellular free water from the brain;[43] it may also reduce the production of CSF.[38] Administration of furosemide in combination with mannitol may reduce ICP more effectively than either drug alone.[9,38,43,49] Roberts et al.[38] showed experimentally that infusion of mannitol followed 15 minutes later by furosemide resulted in the most profound and sustained reduction of elevated ICP. This synergistic effect did not appear to involve altered renal excretion of mannitol. It is also possible that furosemide helps sustain the elevated serum osmolality or the osmotic gradient across the blood-brain barrier induced by mannitol.[38] At present, furosemide is advocated as potentially useful by some in the treatment of elevated ICP after head injury.[8,23] In combination, however, furosemide and mannitol may cause rapid dehydration, which can be harmful to the head-injured patient.

Barbiturates

Barbiturate coma is another way to treat otherwise intractable elevations in ICP.[8,28,33,46,48] Barbiturates reduce ICP by lowering cerebral metabolism and blood flow.[8,28,46] The systemic hypotension that commonly follows barbiturate administration[8,46,48] can be managed with arterial and Swan-Ganz catheters to aid fluid administration and with cardiac pressors, such as dopamine, to maintain adequate cardiac output. In a recent multicenter trial, high-dose barbiturates reduced ICP among patients whose ICP remained above 25 mm Hg despite maximal conventional therapy, including sedation, hyperventilation, and mannitol infusion.[10] Although barbiturates lower ICP, their effect on outcome is less clear.[8,46,48] In a randomized, controlled, prospective trial of barbiturate coma for severe head injury regardless of ICP, Ward et al.[48] showed that there was no improvement in survival and no difference in the incidence or duration of elevated ICP. Although their benefits appear to be limited, barbiturates have a role in the treatment of severely head-injured patients with elevated ICP unresponsive to other therapy.

Additional Measures

Sedation alone may prevent restlessness, frequent posturing, and vigorous movement in response to stimulation, which often increase ICP in head-injured patients with poor intracranial compliance.[8] For this purpose, we use small doses of morphine sulfate (1–3 mg/hr IV) or diazepam (5–10 mg/3–4 hr IM) and avoid sedatives that exert a potentially prolonged or irreversible effect on the central nervous system, such as barbiturates. In addition, we elevate the head of the patient's bed approximately 20° to enhance venous drainage and lower venous pressure.[33]

Management of Arterial Blood Pressure

Continuous monitoring of arterial blood pressure to prevent or correct hypotension or excessive hypertension and maintain an adequate CPP is as important as controlling elevated ICP. Systemic hypotension alone can cause ischemic brain injury. If the blood pressure is unstable, we insert a central venous pressure (CVP) catheter via the jugular or upper extremity veins to monitor the CVP and to administer fluids.[45]

Intravascular volume should be adjusted to maintain or stabilize the systolic blood pressure above 100 mm Hg. If the blood pressure is stable from the outset, fluid resuscitation should be judicious to prevent overhydration, which may augment cerebral edema[45] and possibly lead to pulmonary edema, especially if there is an associated pulmonary contusion. If present, shock must be reversed as quickly and effectively as possible.[20]

Hemorrhagic or hypovolemic shock is most common in trauma patients.[20,45] In patients with multiple injuries, there may be additional causes of shock, such as a low cardiac output due to cardiac contusion or cardiac tamponade or a loss of peripheral vascular tone due to an injury of the cervical spinal cord. It is important to consider these additional causes of shock, especially if the blood pressure does not respond to initial volume resuscitation. Absolute blood pressure may be a less accurate measure of shock than pulse rate, skin perfusion, and urine output because compensatory mechanisms may allow blood pressure to remain relatively stable during hemorrhage until profound volume loss causes it to fall abruptly.

At San Francisco General Hospital, balanced salt (crystalloid) solutions, such as lactated Ringer's solution, are used for initial volume expansion.[6] Replacement of depleted extracellular fluid with lactated Ringer's solution has a significant benefit in the cellular and clinical response to shock.[6] Although colloidal solutions have been used to treat shock or increased ICP, crystalloid solutions appear to have similar hemodynamic and pulmonary effects if given to the same hemodynamic end point.[20] Crystalloid solutions, however, tend to equilibrate more rapidly into the interstitial space and therefore a greater volume will be required. Experimental data suggest that increased serum glucose and intravenous glucose infusion may harm injured and ischemic brain.[35,36] Therefore, crystalloid solutions with added glucose should be avoided unless hypoglycemia is documented.

If repeated measurements show a decreasing hematocrit, cross-matched, packed red blood cells should be transfused. Use of whole blood is indicated if additional volume is needed to support the blood pressure. To ensure optimal perfusion and oxygen carrying capacity, the hematocrit should be approximately 32%–35%.[20] All solutions and blood should be warmed before infusion to avoid causing cardiac arrhythmias from rapid infusion of cold fluids.[45]

Because cerebral autoregulation often is abnormal after severe head injury, systolic hypertension alone may result in an excessive increase in CBF and volume, and thus ICP.[8,39,40] The hemodynamic pattern commonly seen after isolated severe head injury suggests increased sympathetic activity. Such patients are generally hypertensive and have tachycardia, increased cardiac output, and low or normal systemic vascular resistance; arterial epinephrine and norepinephrine levels are elevated.[39,40] The systolic blood pressure should be reduced to less than 160 mm Hg to prevent excessive increase in cerebral blood volume. Beta-adrenergic blockers, such as propranolol, are most effective in treating hypertension and normalizing the hemodynamic pattern seen in severe head injury.[40] Newer short-acting beta-blockers, such as esmolol, administered as a continuous intravenous infusion provide excellent control of blood pressure and allow rapid titration of dosage and effect.[14]

Nutritional Management

After any major trauma, including severe head injury, a negative nitrogen balance may develop rapidly. Aggressive intake of both calories and protein is required to avoid significant weight loss and muscle atrophy.[13,30] Inadequate nutrition may result in impaired immune function, poor wound healing, anemia, and decreased resistance to infection.[13] After severe head injury, enteral feeding may be poorly tolerated initially because of prolonged paralytic ileus, abdominal distention, and diarrhea.[30] Norton et al.[30] showed that the mean delay until adequate volumes of full strength enteral nutrition could be given was 11.5 days after admission; tolerance to feeding was inversely related to the development of increased ICP. They recommended that total parenteral nutrition (TPN) should be started soon after admission. In a prospective, randomized, controlled trial of patients with acute head injury, Rapp et al.[34] showed improved survival in patients who received early TPN compared with enterally fed controls. In a similar study, Hadley et al.[12] found no difference in survival among patients randomized to parenteral or enteral nutrition, although nitrogen balance was significantly better among patients who received TPN.

The complications associated with TPN led Hodge[13] and others[11] to recommend that enteral feedings be attempted as early as 24 to 48 hours after injury. They used continuous enteral infusion of a formula containing 2 kcal/ml, with a goal of providing 100–150 ml/hr. We generally attempt early institution of enteral feeding; for patients with gastric retention we have used a feeding tube passed directly into the jejunum. TPN has been reserved for patients with a prolonged intolerance to enteral feeding or with abdominal injuries that prevent enteral feeding initially.

Metabolic Management

Because metabolic complications are common after severe head injury, we monitor serum electrolytes and osmolality every 6 hours for the first 48 hours of ICU management, and less frequently if the clinical condition has stabilized. The most common metabolic abnormalities stem from electrolyte imbalance, specifically hyper- and hyponatremia.[11,33] Hypernatremia and a hyperosmolar state may result from the frequent use of mannitol and diuretic therapy and from restricting free water intake to prevent or decrease cerebral edema. Excessive hypernatremia can cause neural dysfunction as well as cardiopulmonary and renal complications.[33] Because it is usually associated with excessive volume depletion, hypernatremia is treated by judicious intravenous volume expansion with hypotonic crystalloid solutions, such as 0.45% normal saline. Serum electrolytes are monitored at least twice daily during treatment.

Water intoxication and abnormally low serum sodium levels may occur as a result of the syndrome of inappropriate antidiuretic hormone secretion (SIADH), or cerebral salt wasting.[2,11,21,33] The criteria for diagnosing SIADH are shown in Table 2. Excessive hyponatremia may increase cerebral edema and ICP and can cause seizures. SIADH may appear several days after injury and result in delayed deterioration. Generally, limiting fluid intake to about 1,000 ml/day is the treatment of choice, but dehydration should be avoided.[11]

Diabetes insipidus, with excessive (>200 ml/hr) and dilute (spe-

Table 11-2 Diagnostic Criteria for the Syndrome of Inappropriate Antidiuretic Hormone Secretion

Serum sodium <135 mEq/l
Serum osmolality <280 mosmol/l
Urine sodium >25 mEq/l
Urine osmolality >100 mosmol/l
Absence of cardiac, renal, or hepatic failure
Absence of thyroid disease
Absence of clinical dehydration or peripheral edema

cific gravity <1.0005) urine output and progressive hypernatremia, may occur as a result of hypothalamic or pituitary injury but is more commonly seen when brain death causes loss of hypothalamic function. Seemingly excessive urine output during initial ICU management often represents a diuresis of excess fluids given during the initial resuscitation. Unlike diabetes insipidus, this does not produce hypernatremia.

Hyperglycemia is common after head injury and may be exacerbated by enteral or parenteral feeding. Serum glucose should be closely monitored and managed by reducing glucose administration or, in severe cases, by administering insulin.

Management of Infections

Pulmonary and urinary infections are the most common infectious complications of acute head injury; those related to the cranial injury itself, such as meningitis, brain abscess, and subdural empyema, are less common.[11,15] Pneumonia results from the inability to clear secretions, the loss of normal mechanics, such as coughing and sighing, and prolonged endotracheal intubation. In our institution, patients who are intubated longer than 5 days often develop pneumonia. Urinary tract infections are usually caused by bladder catheterization. Both sources of infection should be assessed periodically, and appropriate cultures should be taken when clinical signs indicate possible infection.

Intracranial infections result either from direct intracranial contamination due to injury or surgery or from a cranial defect, such as skull fracture with leakage of CSF.[15] Occasionally, no obvious source of contamination is found. Such complications may cause delayed neurological deterioration and must be considered when such deterioration is documented. A question which sometimes arises is the safety of performing a lumbar puncture for CSF studies and culture in patients with possible mass lesions. Lumbar puncture in such cases may cause downward herniation of the brain through the tentorial notch or foramen magnum and further neurological deterioration or death. Generally, we rely on a current CT scan to determine the presence of an intracranial mass lesion; lumbar puncture is avoided if a significant mass or obvious radiographic signs of elevated ICP are present.

Although we administer prophylactic antibiotics (cephalexin, 1 g IV) if surgery is performed, in general we do not advocate the use of prophylactic antibiotics for head injury. They have not been shown to provide benefit, and may select for intracranial infection with more resistant bacterial strains.

References

1. Andrews BT: Management of delayed post-traumatic intracerebral hemorrhage. Contemp Neurosurg 10:1-6, 1988.
2. Andrews BT, Fitzgerald PA, Tyrell JB, et al.: Cerebral salt-wasting after pituitary exploration and biopsy. Case report. Neurosurgery 18:469-471, 1986.
3. Andrews BT, Pitts LH, Lovely MP, et al.: Is computed tomographic scanning necessary in patients with tentorial herniation? Results of immediate surgical exploration without computed tomography in 100 patients. Neurosurgery 19:408-413, 1986.
4. Bruce DA, Alavi A, Bilanuik L, et al.: Diffuse cerebral swelling following head injuries in children. The syndrome of "malignant brain edema." J Neurosurg 55:170-178, 1981.
5. Burke AM, Quest DO, Chien S, et al.: The effects of mannitol on blood viscosity. J Neurosurg 55:550-553, 1981.
6. Canizaro PC, Prager MD, Shires GT: The infusion of Ringer's lactate solution during shock. Changes in lactate, excess lactate, and pH. Am J Surg 122:494-501, 1971.
7. Christensen MS: Acid-base changes in cerebrospinal fluid and blood, and blood volume changes following prolonged hyperventilation in man. Br J Anaesth 46:348-357, 1974.
8. Clifton GL: Management of elevated intracranial pressure. Neurology Clinics, Baylor College of Medicine 4:25-29, 1982.
9. Cottrell JE, Robustelli A, Post K: Furosemide and mannitol induced changes in intracranial pressure and serum osmolality and electrolytes. Anesthesiology 47:28-30, 1977.
10. Eisenberg HM, Frankowski RF, Conant CF, et al.: High-dose barbiturate control of elevated intracranial pressure in patients with severe head injury. J Neurosurg 69:15-23, 1988.
11. Epstein FM, Ward JD, Becker DP: Medical complications of head injury. In Cooper PR (ed): Head Injury. 2nd ed. Baltimore, MD: Williams & Wilkins, 1987, pp 390-421.

12. Hadley MN, Grahm TW, Harrington T, et al.: Nutritional support and neurotrauma. A critical review of early nutritional support in forty-five acute head injury patients. Neurosurgery 19:367-373, 1986.
13. Hodge SH: Nutritional management. Neurology Clinics, Baylor College of Medicine 4:34-35, 1982.
14. Kaplan JA (ed): Esmolol and the Adrenergic Response to Perioperative Stimuli. Proceedings from a Symposium, San Francisco, October 13, 1985. New York: Biomedical Information Corporation, 1986, 62 pp.
15. Landesman S, Rechtman D, Cooper PR: Infectious complications of head injury. In Cooper PR (ed): Head Injury. 2nd ed. Baltimore, MD: Williams & Wilkins, 1987, pp 422-441.
16. Langfitt TW: Increased intracranial pressure and the cerebral circulation. In Youmans JR (ed): Neurological Surgery. Philadelphia, PA: WB Saunders, 1982, pp 846-930.
17. Lassen NA: The luxury-perfusion syndrome and its possible relation to acute metabolic acidosis localized within the brain. Lancet 2:1113-1115, 1966.
18. Lassen NA: Brain extracellular pH. The main factor controlling cerebral blood flow. Scand J Clin Lab Invest 22:247-251, 1968.
19. Leech PJ, Miller JD: Intracranial volume-pressure relationships during experimental brain compression in primates. Part 3. The effect of mannitol and hypocapnia. J Neurol Neurosurg Psychiatry 37:1105-1111, 1974.
20. Lewis FR: Initial assessment and resuscitation: Symposium on Multiple Trauma. Emerg Med Clin North Am 2:733-748, 1984.
21. Lester MC, Nelson PB: Neurological aspects of vasopressin release and the syndrome of inappropriate secretion of antidiuretic hormone. Neurosurgery 8:735-740, 1981.
22. Lundberg N, Kjallquist A, Bien C: Reduction of increased intracranial pressure by hyperventilation. Acta Psychiatr Scand 34 (Suppl) 139:1-64, 1959.
23. Marshall LF, Marshall SB: Medical management of intracranial pressure. In Cooper PR (ed): Head Injury. 2nd ed. Baltimore, MD: Williams & Wilkins, 1987, pp 177-196.
24. Muizelaar JP, Lutz HA, Becker DP: Effect of mannitol on ICP and CBF and correlation with pressure autoregulation in severely head-injured patients. J Neurosurg 61:700-706, 1984.
25. Muizlaar JP, van der Poel HG, Li Z, et al.: Pial arteriolar vessel

diameter and CO_2 reactivity during prolonged hyperventilation in the rabbit. J Neurosurg 69:923-927, 1988.
26. Muizlaar JP, Wei EP, Kontos HA, et al.: Mannitol causes compensatory cerebral vasoconstriction and vasodilatation in response to blood viscosity changes. J Neurosurg 59:822-828, 1983.
27. Narayan RK, Kishore PR, Becker DP, et al.: Intracranial pressure: To monitor or not to monitor? A review of our experience with severe head injury. J Neurosurg 56:650-659, 1982.
28. Nordstrom CH, Messeter K, Sundbarg G, et al.: Cerebral blood flow, vasoreactivity and oxygen consumption during barbiturate therapy in severe traumatic brain lesions. J Neurosurg 68:424-431, 1988.
29. North B, Reilly P: Comparison among three methods of intracranial pressure recording. Neurosurgery 18:730-732, 1986.
30. Norton JA, Ott LG, McClain C, et al.: Intolerance to enteral feeding in the brain-injured patient. J Neurosurg 68:62-66, 1988.
31. Ostrup RC, Luerssen TG, Marshall LF, et al.: Continuous monitoring of intracranial pressure with a miniaturized fiberoptic device. J Neurosurg 67:206-209, 1987.
32. Paul RL, Polanco O, Turney SZ, et al.: Intracranial pressure responses to alterations in arterial carbon dioxide pressure in patients with head injuries. J Neurosurg 36:714-720, 1972.
33. Pitts LH, Martin N: Head injuries. Surg Clin North Am 62:47-60, 1982.
34. Rapp RP, Young B, Twyman D, et al.: The favorable effect of early parenteral feeding on survival in head-injured patients. J Neurosurg 58:906-912, 1983.
35. Rehncrona S, Rosen I, Siesjö B: Excessive cellular acidosis: an important mechanism of neuronal damage in the brain. Acta Physiol Scand 110:435-437, 1980.
36. Rehncrona S, Rosen I, Siesjö B: Brain lactic acidosis and ischemic cell damage. 1: Biochemistry and neurophysiology. J Cereb Blood Flow Metab 1:297-311, 1981.
37. Reivich M: Arterial pco_2 and cerebral hemodynamics. Am J Physiol 206:25-35, 1964.
38. Roberts PA, Pollay M, Engles C, et al.: Effect on intracranial pressure of furosemide combined with varying doses and administration of mannitol. J Neurosurg 66:440-446, 1987.

39. Robertson CS: The cardiovascular profile of head injury. Neurology Clinics, Baylor College of Medicine 4:30-33, 1982.
40. Robertson CS, Clifton JL, Taylor AA, et al.: Treatment of hypertension associated with head injury. J Neurosurg 59:455-460, 1983.
41. Rosner MJ, Coley I: Cerebral perfusion pressure: A hemodynamic mechanism of mannitol and the postmannitol hemogram. Neurosurgery 21:147-156, 1987.
42. Saul TG: Acute head injuries in adults. In Rakel RE (ed): Conn's Current Therapy. 38th ed. Philadelphia, PA: WB Saunders, 1987, pp 776-782.
43. Schettini A, Stahurski B, Young HF: Osmotic and osmotic-loop diuresis in brain surgery. Effects on plasma and CSF electrolytes and ion secretion. J Neurosurg 56:679-684, 1982.
44. Teasdale G, Jennett B: Assessment of coma and impaired consciousness. Lancet 2:81-84, 1974.
45. Thal ER: Initial management of the multiply injured patient. In Cooper PR (ed): Head Injury. 2nd ed. Baltimore, MD: Williams & Wilkins, 1987, pp 34-50.
46. Trauner DA: Barbiturate therapy in acute brain injury. J Pediatr 109:742-746, 1986.
47. Tsutsumi H, Ide K, Mizutani T, et al.: The relationship between intracranial pressure, cerebral perfusion pressure and outcome in head-injured patient. The critical level of cerebral perfusion pressure. In Miller JD, Teasdale GM, Rowan JO, et al. (eds): Intracranial Pressure VI. Berlin: Springer-Verlag, 1985, pp 661-666.
48. Ward JD, Becker DP, Miller JD, et al.: Failure of prophylactic barbiturate coma in the treatment of severe head injury. J Neurosurg 62:383-388, 1985.
49. Wilkinson HA, Wepsic JG, Austin G: Diuretic synergy in the treatment of acute experimental cerebral edema. J Neurosurg 34:203-208, 1971.
50. Winn HR, Dacey RG, Jane JA: Intracranial subarachnoid pressure recording. Experience with 650 patients. Surg Neurol 8:41-47, 1977.
51. Wise BL, Chater N: The value of hypertonic mannitol solution in decreasing brain mass and lowering cerebrospinal fluid pressure. J Neurosurg 19:1038-1043, 1962.

CHAPTER 12

Post-Traumatic Sequelae and Rehabilitation

The outcome after severe head injury has usually been evaluated by assessing motor function and the level of independence. Less obvious cognitive and intellectual abnormalities[9,21] and other forms of persistent morbidity have generally been overlooked or disregarded. Recently there has been increasing recognition of the more subtle neurological, cognitive, and psychological deficits that may cause significant long-term disability, even among patients without residual sensorimotor deficits.[13,19,24,27,28,34,36] For the physician, the cognitive and behavioral sequelae of severe head injury are difficult to diagnose and treat; for patients and their families, they are often more difficult to cope with than residual focal neurological deficits.

In this chapter, we describe some of the subjective symptoms that may persist after head injury, including postconcussion syndrome and traumatic epilepsy, and discuss their management. We also review the cognitive and psychosocial sequelae of head injury and methods for their diagnosis and treatment.

The "Postconcussion" Syndrome

Persistent physical complaints may occur after any grade of head trauma, from a minor injury with brief loss of consciousness to severe injury with major residual neurological deficits. These symptoms

From *Traumatic Transtentorial Herniation and Its Management* by Brian T. Andrews, MD and Lawrence H. Pitts, MD © 1991, Futura Publishing Co., Inc., Mount Kisco, NY.

usually remain unnoticed while the patient recovers from major deficits in level of consciousness and the systemic effects and complications of trauma. With further recovery, however, the patient becomes more aware of subjective symptoms, including headache, dizziness, nausea and vomiting, and alcohol intolerance;[12,19,24,28,35] additional complaints may include anxiety, irritability, changes in personality, and difficulties with concentration and memory. We refer to this constellation of symptoms as the postconcussion syndrome.

Perhaps the most common symptom of postconcussion syndrome is persistent headache, which is present in up to 93% of patients 3 months after moderately severe head injury.[19] Although variable in character and duration, postconcussion headaches are typically diffuse and may be aggravated by movement, change of position, anxiety, or stress. They are frequently accompanied by dizziness, nausea, vomiting, and insomnia.[19,24,28,35]

Traumatic dizziness is also very common. It may initially be described as a pronounced vertigo that is exacerbated by movement or changes in position, and is frequently associated with nausea. The dizziness may be followed by intermittent unsteadiness, which is often positional or made worse by movement, and adds to mobility problems caused by hemiparesis or sensory loss. These symptoms tend to resolve over the course of weeks to months after injury.[35]

There is some evidence that the duration and severity of postconcussion symptoms are directly related to the severity of the head injury.[19,24,34,36] Long-lasting symptoms most often occur in patients with persistent focal neurological deficits or an intracranial hematoma.[24] The actual cause of postconcussive symptoms, however, is unknown. Psychological disturbance, compensation, litigation, and malingering have been proposed,[24] but recent evidence indicates that structural abnormalities are a more likely cause.[19]

In about 50% of patients with dizziness after minor or moderate head injury, electronystagmographic testing shows abnormalities; auditory evoked potentials in these patients show prolonged mean latencies that suggest structural abnormalities of the brain stem.[35] Diffuse structural injury, including neuronal loss and microscopic lesions in the pyramidal tracts of the medulla and pons, is often found at autopsy after severe head injury.[19,32,33] Magnetic resonance (MR) imaging has shown a variety of structural abnormalities in frontal and temporal regions or in the brain stem of patients after head injury, even though computed tomography (CT) scans may appear normal.[26,44] Subarachnoid bleeding at the time of injury may lead to meningeal irritation or subsequent abnormalities of CSF flow, with increased intracranial pressure. Stretching and tearing of vascular or dural attachments of the brain may also engender painful sequelae. Pain from scalp injury or neuralgia from the supraorbital or occipital nerves may occasionally play a role in postconcussive headaches.[24]

Treatment

Treatment of postconcussion syndrome has primarily been directed toward alleviating symptoms. For headaches, we initially prescribe acetaminophen with 30 mg of codeine every 3–4 hours. Treatment usually begins during hospitalization or after the initial evaluation. Propoxyphene (Darvon), 32–65 mg every 3–6 hours, may also be used; although it is less effective than codeine, it is also somewhat less addictive.[17] After 1 to 2 weeks, an attempt is made to wean the patient to a nonopiate compound, such as acetaminophen, 650 mg every 4–6 hours; ibuprofen, 400–800 mg three times daily; or another nonsteroidal anti-inflammatory analgesic.

Dizziness that appears to be vertiginous may respond to vestibular suppressants. We have used the antihistamine meclizine (Antivert), 25–50 mg four times daily as needed, with good results; diphenhydramine (Benadryl) at the same dose and schedule may also be used. The side effects of antihistamines are somnolence and mental dullness.

Nausea and vomiting should be treated only after it has been determined that they do not stem from persistently increased intracranial pressure caused by a delayed complication, such as an intracerebral hemorrhage or enlarging chronic subdural hematoma. This is particularly important in patients who have worsening headaches or who have a delayed onset of postconcussion symptoms. Several medications may be effective. Antihistamines, such as diphenhydramine, 25–50 mg four times daily, suppress nausea centrally and may prove to be adequate. The phenothiazine prochlorperazine (Compazine), 25 mg, given in suppository form twice daily is a potent centrally acting antiemetic; however, it lowers the seizurethreshold and may be contraindicated for patients at risk for traumatic seizures. Phenothiazines also increase mental dullness, which may be particularly disturbing in head-injured patients with neuropsychological sequelae.

Sleep disturbance may be treated with a variety of agents, but treatment should be delayed by several weeks to a month or more after injury to avoid masking the clinical signs of a delayed complication, such as intracerebral hemorrhage. We initially prescribe diphenhydramine, 25–50 mg at bedtime, which acts as a mild sedative. The benzodiazepine compound flurazepam (Dalmane), 15–30 mg, is an effective hypnotic but has undesirable side effects, including excessive morning drowsiness, vertigo, ataxia, and falling,[18] which may make this drug inappropriate for patients with unsteadiness or focal neurological deficits. The shorter-acting benzodiazepines temazepam (Restoril), 15–30 mg, and triazolam (Halcion), 0.125–0.25 mg, have been used as night-time sedatives. Although they cause less residual morning drowsiness, these drugs have side effects similar to those of other benzodiazepines. Generally, benzodiazepines should be prescribed for no more than approximately 3 weeks to prevent habituation.[18]

Traumatic Epilepsy

Traumatic epilepsy occurs in a significant number of head-injured patients. Early epilepsy, the term used by Jennett and Teasdale to describe seizures occurring within 7 days after injury, occurs in approximately 5% of patients after blunt trauma.[23,24] Early epilepsy is most common after penetrating injury[4] and severe trauma resulting in depressed skull fractures, focal neurological deficits, and intracranial hematomas; it is also more frequent in young children than in adults.[22] Without anticonvulsant therapy, approximately 42% of patients with penetrating injuries have early seizures;[4] Apuzzo et al.[38] reported that 10% of patients with gunshot wounds of the brain had early epilepsy despite the routine use of anticonvulsants.

Delayed traumatic epilepsy, defined as seizures occurring more than 7 days after injury, occurs in approximately 5% of all patients with closed head trauma.[7,11,23] Approximately 15% of adults with depressed skull fractures, 25% of those with early epilepsy, and 35% of those with intracranial hematomas develop persistent seizures.[11]

The combination of prolonged traumatic amnesia or coma, depressed skull fracture, and a focal brain injury, such as an intracerebral hematoma, increases the risk of delayed epilepsy to as high as 70%. The occurrence of a seizure more than 7 days after injury increases the risk of further epilepsy to at least 75%.[11] Seventy percent of traumatic seizures are grand mal, 10% are partial seizures without loss of consciousness, and 20% are complex partial seizures.[23]

Although more than 50% of delayed seizures occur within 12 months after injury, a first seizure may occur even years later. Among 481 patients with delayed epilepsy studied by Jennett, 27% had their first seizure within 3 months and 56% within 1 year after injury. Thereafter, the frequency of seizures decreased each year. In 25% of patients, however, the onset was delayed 4 years or more.[20,23] Patients with delayed epilepsy remain at risk for further seizures. Seizures may recur after temporary remissions of as long as 2 years.[3,20,23] For this reason it has been recommended that anticonvulsant therapy be continued indefinitely in patients with delayed epilepsy, even years after successful therapy.

Treatment

For patients who appear to be at risk of developing traumatic seizures, prophylactic therapy may begin at admission.[7] Factors that increase the risk of seizures include subdural or intraparenchymal hematomas, significant parenchymal contusions, depressed skull fractures,[11] and penetrating dural injury causing cortical laceration.[4,38] Others have recommended prophylactic anticonvulsant therapy for any patient with a severe head injury, regardless of the degree of obvious cortical injury.[11] All head-injured patients who have had a seizure, except infants with early seizures, should receive anticonvulsant therapy. The most frequently used drug is phenytoin (Dilantin), which is given first as a loading dose, 15 mg/kg intravenously. To avoid myocardial suppression, which could lead to systemic hypotension, phenytoin must not be infused at a rate exceeding 50 mg/min; an even slower rate should be used for elderly patients.[46] The subsequent oral or intravenous dosage is 3–4 mg/kg per day; serum drug levels should be monitored to achieve the optimal therapeutic level of 10–20 μg/ml. The side effects of phenytoin include nystagmus, ataxia, behavioral changes, hirsutism, coarsening of facial features, gingival hyperplasia, gastrointestinal symptoms, and rash.[7,46] Phenobarbital and carbamazepine (Tegretol) are both effective for generalized seizures[29] but can cause central nervous system depression, and therefore may not be well-tolerated by head-injured patients.

The duration of anticonvulsant therapy is somewhat controversial. Deutschman and Haines suggest that prophylactic therapy should be continued if the risk of persistent seizures is 15% or greater.[7] This would include patients with early or delayed traumatic seizures, depressed skull fractures, subdural or intraparenchymal hematomas, and penetrating injury with dural and cortical lacerations.[7] We prescribe anticonvulsants for 6 months to 1 year for patients with minimal cortical injury or subdural hematomas who have not had seizures. Patients who have had a delayed seizure and those at high risk for persistent seizures, including patients with penetrating cortical trauma, gunshot wounds, and significant focal cortical injury, are maintained on anticonvulsant therapy indefinitely. Others have suggested that anticonvulsant therapy may be discontinued among higher-risk patients who have not had seizures for 1 to 2 years and whose EEGs show no paroxysmal abnormalities.[11]

Cognitive Sequelae of Severe Head Injury

Numerous studies have documented the profound cognitive sequelae of severe head injury.[10,24,27,41] In patients who were alert soon after severe head injury, Tabaddor et al.[41] found global impairment of intellectual function, particularly memory. No differences were found between patients who had an operation and those who did not. Patients with focal lesions in the dominant hemisphere had greater impairment in verbal IQ, whereas those with lesions of the nondominant hemisphere had greater impairment of performance IQ.[41] Others have also shown similar initial deficits among the severely head injured.[10,24] One year after injury, further testing showed improvement, but cognitive deficits, specifically of language and memory, remained significant. The cognitive outcome was predicted by the patient's age, initial Glasgow coma score, and how soon after injury the patient could follow simple two-step commands.[41] Levin et al.[25] have also documented persistent deficits of memory, language, and social adjustment one year after severe head injury. In general, these deficits reflected the overall outcome. That is, patients with good overall outcome had mild cognitive deficits; patients with moderate disabilities had significant deficits, primarily of performance IQ and memory; and patients with severe disability had profound global intellectual impairment and were the only group to have persistent anomia and dysphasia. While repetition led to progressive gains in memory among patients who had a good outcome, those with a moderately severe deficit showed less improvement, and those with a persistent severe disability improved very little. Patients with abnormal oculocephalic reflexes often had prolonged cognitive and neuropsychological impairment.[25,27]

Persistent cognitive deficits after severe head injury are probably caused in part by the effects of shear injury to the brain at multiple levels, including the grey and white matter junction of the cortex, the midbrain, and lower parts of the brain stem. Shear forces stretch and disrupt axons and cause secondary neural degeneration.[19,32] In moderately severe experimental head injury, diffuse degeneration of axons occurs in the subcortical white matter.[19] Similar abnormalities are seen in humans at autopsy after head injury.[33]

Uzzell et al.[42] reported that abnormalities on initial CT scans predicted the extent of neuropsychological impairment and recovery after severe head injury. Levels of memory and learning were initially highest among patients with CT evidence of diffuse swelling only. Patients with evidence of diffuse axonal injury (midline hemorrhages and small hemorrhages at the gray-white junction) had greater initial impairment, but also improved more than the other groups. Patients with unilateral intracerebral hemorrhages and contusions had the greatest disability and least improvement in recall and learning.[42] MR imaging has demonstrated diffuse abnormalities in the white matter and brain stem that were not apparent on CT scans of patients with severe head injury.[25,44]

In addition to shear injury,[19,32] there may be additional diffuse brain injury from hypotension, hypoxia,[30] or increased intracranial pressure[31] as well as focal injuries, such as contusions,[6] intracranial hematomas,[40] and brain stem compression resulting from transtentorial herniation.[1]

The location of focal brain injury may determine the type of cognitive deficits after head trauma. Eisenberg et al.[10] reported that patients with traumatic lesions of the left temporal lobe had much more severe initial deficits of verbal memory, similar to those of patients with diffuse or bilateral lesions, than patients with focal lesions in other areas. However, recovery of verbal memory was much greater in patients with left temporal lesions than in those with diffuse injury and may have involved increased participation of the nondominant hemisphere.[10] Recent evidence suggests that the right hemisphere may be dominant for spatial attention;[43] if so, injury to the right hemisphere may lead to bilateral cognitive deficits involving spatial relationships and performance tasks. MR imaging has also demonstrated localized abnormalities in the white matter and brain stem that are not apparent on CT scans of severely head-injured patients.[25,44] These lesions probably correlate with specific cognitive deficits in severely head-injured patients, as has already been established in patients with mild and moderately severe head injuries.[26]

Psychosocial and Behavioral Sequelae

Psychosocial and behavioral sequelae may occur regardless of the severity of the head injury. These symptoms may have a profound impact on patients and their families. Depression, withdrawal, and anxiety[8,28] are common; in addition, affective symptoms, including increased aggressiveness and hostility,[27] can become as severe as full-blown mania[39] or psychosis.[27] Patients recovering from severe head injury often fail to appreciate the severity of their cognitive deficits, which can have a negative influence on their behavior. Increased irritability, indifference, confabulations, delusions and aggressiveness have been described.[25] Such patients have a marked tendency to become socially isolated, and may display frankly psychotic symptoms requiring hospitalization.[27] Interviews with relatives of severely head-injured patients indicate that the behavioral sequelae of the head injury are often more difficult to cope with than residual cognitive or focal neurological deficits, and that these difficulties have not diminished by one year after injury.[25]

Cognitive and Psychosocial Rehabilitation

One of the major challenges in the rehabilitation of head-injured patients is to improve neuropsychological deficits, especially cognitive deficits, such as attention and memory. Wood has significantly improved attention-to-task by use of positive reinforcement (reward).[45] The use of electronic and computerized training methods to improve focusing and attention span has resulted in gains on psychometric tests and and in functional skills.[15] The use of mnemonics, visual imagery, and verbal and procedural strategies for storing and retrieving information to improve memory have met with little or mixed success among the severely head-injured because of the mental effort they require. These techniques may be more beneficial among less impaired patients.[14] External aids such as notebooks, lists, calculators, and computers, cuing devices such as alarm clocks, and structured environments that reduce memory load may be useful but have not been systematically evaluated beyond the acute rehabilitation setting.[16]

Another area of current interest is the reintegration of brain-injured children and adolescents into the educational system. Because of their cognitive and behavioral deficits, moderately and severely injured patients generally cannot return to their previous school. The Education for All Handicapped Children's Act of 1975 focused attention on developing specialized academic and adaptive-behavioral strategies and vocational-rehabilitation counseling within the school system to allow successful reintegration of children and adolescents. Similar efforts in postsecondary and vocational education have been made for head-injured adults.[37] Ben-Yishay et al.[2] have shown that application of an intensive outpatient program emphasizing cognitive, behavioral, and vocational rehabilitation results in successful employability or productivity of 84% of previously unemployable head-injured adults.

To successfully reintegrate the head-injured patient into society after inpatient rehabilitation is complete, the family and community setting into which the patient is placed must be evaluated. The evaluation addresses the difficulties the family may face in dealing with the behavioral changes and dependency of the patient. Subsequent guidance and instruction are tailored to meet the specific needs of the individual patient and family.[5]

It is clear that rehabilitation efforts aimed at the specific cognitive deficits and psychosocial problems in severely head-injured patients are only now being explored. These efforts are occurring primarily in the outpatient setting and focus on reintegrating the patient into the community. We can only hope for an improvement in cognitive recovery and in psychosocial and vocational capabilities as these methods become more refined and available.

References

1. Andrews BT, Pitts LH, Lovely MP, et al.: Is CT scanning necessary in patients with tentorial herniation: results of immediate surgical exploration without CT scanning in 100 patients. Neurosurgery 19:408-413, 1986.
2. Ben-Yishay Y, Silver SM, Piasetsky E, et al.: Relationship between employability and vocational outcome after intensive holistic cognitive rehabilitation. J Head Trauma Rehabil 2:35-48, 1987.
3. Caveness WF: Onset and cessation of fits following craniocerebral trauma. J Neurosurg 20:570-583, 1963.
4. Caveness WF, Liss HR: Incidence of post-traumatic epilepsy. Epilepsia 2:123-129, 1961.
5. Condeluci A, Gretz-Lasky S: Social role valorization: a model for community reentry. J Head Trauma Rehabil 2:49-56, 1987.
6. Cooper PR: Post-traumatic intracranial mass lesions. In Cooper PR (ed): Head Injury. 2nd ed. Baltimore, MD: Williams and Wilkins, 1987, pp 238-284.
7. Deutschmann CS, Haines SJ: Anticonvulsant prophylaxis in neurological surgery. Neurosurgery 17:510-517, 1985.
8. Dikmen S, Reitan R: Emotional sequelae of head injury. Ann Neurol 2:492-494, 1977.
9. Eisenberg HM: Outcome after head injury: general considerations and neurobehavioral recovery. Part 1: general considerations. In Becker DP, Povlishock JT (eds): Central Nervous System Trauma Status Report. Bethesda, MD: National Institute of Neurological and Communicative Disorders and Stroke, National Institutes of Health, 1985, pp 271-280.
10. Eisenberg HM, Levin HS, Papanicolaou AC: Recovery of memory after head injury. In: Dacey RG, Winn HR, Rimel RW, et al. (eds): Trauma of the Central Nervous System. New York: Raven Press, 1985, pp 35-47.
11. Epstein FM, Ward JD, Becker DP: Medical complications of head injury. In Cooper PR (ed): Head Injury. 2nd ed. Baltimore, MD: Williams and Wilkins, 1987, pp 390-421.

12. Feldman WS: Post-concussive syndrome: what a headache. Legal Aspects of Medical Practice July: 4–6, 1986.
13. Gentilini M, Nichelli P, Schoenhuber R, et al.: Neuropsychological evaluation of mild head injury. J Neurol Neurosurg Psychiatry 48:137-140, 1985.
14. Gilsky EL, Schacter DL: Remediation of organic memory disorders: current status and future prospects. J Head Trauma Rehabil 1:54-63, 1986.
15. Grafman J: Memory assessment and remediation in brain-injured patients. In Edelstein B, Couture EC (eds): Behavior Assessment and Treatment of the Traumatically Brain Damaged. New York: Plenum Press, 1983.
16. Harris J: Methods of improving memory. In Wilson BA, Moffat N (eds): Clinical Management of Memory Problems. Rockville, MD: Aspen, 1984.
17. Harvey SC: Hypnotics and sedatives. In Goodman LS, Gilman A (eds): The Pharmacologic Basis of Therapeutics. New York: Macmillan, 1975, pp 124-136.
18. Jaffe JH, Martin WR: Narcotic analgesics and antagonists. In Goodman LS, Gilman A (eds): The Pharmacologic Basis of Therapeutics. New York: Macmillan, 1975, pp 245-283.
19. Jane JA, Rimel RW, Alves WM, et al.: Minor and moderate head injury: model systems. In Dacey RG, Winn HR, Rimel RW, et al. (eds): Trauma of the Central Nervous System. New York: Raven Press, 1985, pp 27-33.
20. Jennett B: Anticonvulsant drugs and advice about driving after head injury and intracranial surgery. Br Med J 286:627-628, 1983.
21. Jennett B, Snoek J, Bond MR, et al.: Disability after severe head injury: observations on the use of the Glasgow Outcome Scale. J Neurol Neurosurg Psychiatry 44:285-293, 1981.
22. Jennett B, Teasdale G: Management of head injuries in the acute stage. In Jennett B, Teasdale G (eds): Management of Head Injuries. Philadelphia, PA: F.A. Davis, 1981, pp 211-252.
23. Jennett B, Teasdale G: Neurophysical sequelae. In Jennett B, Teasdale G (eds): Management of Head Injuries. Philadelphia, PA: F.A. Davis, 1981, pp 271-288.
24. Jennett B, Teasdale G: Recovery after head injury. In Jennett B, Teasdale G (eds): Management of Head Injuries. Philadelphia, PA: F.A. Davis, 1981, pp 253-269.

25. Levin HS: Neurobehavioral sequelae of head injury. In Cooper PR (ed): Head Injury. 2nd ed. Baltimore, MD: Williams and Wilkins, 1987, pp 442-463.
26. Levin HS, Amparo E, Eisenberg HM, et al.: Magnetic resonance imaging and computerized tomography in relation to the neurobehavioral sequelae of mild and moderate head injuries. J Neurosurg 66:706-713, 1987.
27. Levin HS, Grossman RG, Rose JE, et al.: Long-term neuropsychological outcome of closed head injury. J Neurosurg 50:412-422, 1979.
28. Levin HS, Mattis S, Ruff RM, et al.: Neurobehavioral outcome following minor head injury. J Neurosurg 66:234-243, 1987.
29. Mattson RH, Cramer JA, Collins JF, et al.: Comparison of carbamazepine, phenobarbital, phenytoin, and primidone in partial and secondarily generalized tonic-clonic seizures. N Engl J Med 313:145-151, 1985.
30. Miller JD, Sweet RC, Narayan R, et al.: Early insults to the injured brain. JAMA 240:439-442, 1978.
31. Narayan RK, Kishore PR, Becker DP, et al.: Intracranial pressure: to monitor or not to monitor? A review of our experience with severe head injury. J Neurosurg 56:650-659, 1982.
32. Ommaya AK, Gennarelli TA: Cerebral concussion and traumatic unconsciousness: correlation of experimental and clinical observations on blunt head injuries. Brain 97:633-654, 1974.
33. Oppenheimer DR: Microscopic lesions in the brain following head injury. J Neurol Neurosurg Psychiatry 31:229-306, 1968.
34. Rimel RW, Giordani B, Barth JT, et al.: Moderate head injury: completing the clinical spectrum of brain trauma. Neurosurgery 11:344-351, 1982.
35. Rowe MJ, Carlson C: Brain stem auditory evoked potentials in postconcussion dizziness. Arch Neurol 37:679-683, 1980.
36. Rutherford WH, Merrett JD, McDonald JR: Sequelae of concussion caused by minor head injury. Lancet 1:1-4, 1977.
37. Savage RC: Educational issues for the head-injured adolescent and young adult. J Head Trauma Rehabil 2:1-10, 1987.
38. Sherman WD, Apuzzo MLJ, Heiden JS: Gunshot wounds to the brain—a civilian experience. West J Med 123:99-105, 1980.
39. Starkstein SE, Pearlson GD, Boston J, et al.: Mania after brain injury: a controlled study of causative factors. Arch Neurol 44: 1069-1073, 1987.

40. Stone JL, Rifai MHS, Sugar O, et al.: Subdural hematomas 1: acute subdural hematomas: progress in definition, clinical pathology, and therapy. Surg Neurol 19:216-231, 1983.
41. Tabaddor K, Mattis S, Zazula T: Cognitive recovery after moderate and severe head injury. In Dacey RG, Winn HR, Rimel RW, et al. (eds): Trauma of the Central Nervous System. New York: Raven Press, 1985, pp 49-63.
42. Uzzell BP, Dolinskas CA, Wiser RF, et al.: Influence of lesions detected by computerized tomography on outcome and neuropsychological recovery after severe head injury. Neurosurgery 20:396-402, 1987.
43. Weintraub S, Mesilam MM: Right cerebral dominance in spatial attention: further evidence based on ipsilateral neglect. Arch Neurol 44:621-625, 1987.
44. Wilberger JE, Deeb Z, Rothfus W: Magnetic resonance imaging in cases of severe head injury. Neurosurgery 20:571-576, 1987.
45. Wood RL: Rehabilitation of patients with disorders of attention. J Head Trauma Rehabil 1:43-53, 1986.
46. Woodbury DM, Fingl E: Drugs effective in the therapy of epilepsies. In Goodman LS, Gilman A (eds): The Pharmacologic Basis of Therapeutics. New York: Macmillan, 1975, pp 201-226.

CHAPTER 13

Prognosis

Although the prognosis for patients with traumatic transtentorial herniation is poor—the mortality rate is about 70% among adults,[7,18–20,37,40,41] and survivors may be left severely disabled or vegetative—it is by no means hopeless. In our series, 9% of patients had a good recovery and 9% were only moderately disabled (see Chapter 7). These patients were generally younger and had a higher initial Glasgow coma score (GCS) than patients who died or were severely disabled or vegetative, and had anisocoria rather than bilaterally dilated pupils. Several had a high GCS that deteriorated with the onset of signs of brain stem dysfunction. Earlier reports, too, have suggested that younger age[1,8,9,13,18,21,30,33,45] and a higher initial GCS[4,6,8,10,12,18,21,33,40,42,50] improve the prognosis. Additional features that influence the potential for recovery include the findings on the initial computerized tomography (CT) scan,[1,5,14,23,46] the presence or absence of intracranial hematomas,[5,8–10,14,15,27,42] and uncontrolled elevations in intracranial pressure (ICP).[9,10,27,29,35,48]

Information on the potential prognosis is important for defining the expectations of the caregivers and family of patients with traumatic transtentorial herniation. Prognostic information also allows realistic discussions with the patient's family concerning treatment, rehabilitation, and organ donation.

From *Traumatic Transtentorial Herniation and Its Management* by Brian T. Andrews, MD and Lawrence H. Pitts, MD © 1991, Futura Publishing Co., Inc., Mount Kisco, NY.

Age

Numerous studies have shown that younger patients have a better outcome than older patients after severe head injury.[1,8,9,13,18,21,24,25,30,33,45] In a review of 1,000 patients divided into 5-year cohorts, Jennett et al.[21] found that mortality and severe morbidity rates increased with age. Becker et al.[8] reported mortality rates of 22% in patients less than 21 years of age and 57% in those over 60 years of age. Gutterman and Shenkin[18] found that older patients were much less able to recover from traumatic decerebration than younger patients. In our series of patients with transtentorial herniation, the mortality rate among children and adolescents (up to 17 years of age) was 45%, and none of the survivors were severely disabled or vegetative (see Chapter 10). Among adults, the mortality rate was 70%, and 12% were severely disabled or vegetative (see Chapter 7). The reasons for the effect of age on outcome include the higher incidence of intracranial hematomas with increasing age[3,7–10,12,13,21,27,42] and the greater likelihood of pre-existing medical conditions in older patients.[3]

Glasgow Coma Score

Perhaps the most significant prognostic variable is the severity of the primary brain injury, which is best reflected by the neurological examinations during the first hours and days.[4,6,8,10,12,18,21,33,40,42,50] The level of consciousness indicated by the highest GCS[44] appears to have a particularly strong influence on survival and the potential for recovery. In the series of Jennett et al.,[21] 82% of patients with a GCS of 11 or more during the first 24 hours had a good recovery or a moderate disability and only 12% were dead or had a severe disability at 6 months. The outcome worsened as the initial GCS decreased; only 7% of patients with a best GCS of 3 or 4 during the first 24 hours had a good outcome or a moderate disability. Numerous other studies have confirmed the relationship between the early GCS and functional outcome.[10,24,50] The early GCS is also a sensitive indicator of the neuropsychological outcome after severe head injury.[2]

In our series, the mean initial GCS among 14 patients (9%) who had a good outcome was 8, and four had an initial score of 12 or more that fell to 8 or less after the onset of clinical signs of upper brain stem compression. The 14 patients (9%) who were moderately disabled had a mean GCS of 6.5; one patient had a high score and later deteriorated. Among patients who died or were severely disabled, the initial mean GCS was 4.3 (see Chapter 7).

Patients who have a high GCS and then deteriorate have a high incidence of intracranial mass lesions.[7,37,39] Although it would seem logical that rapid diagnosis and evacuation of the mass would increase the chance of a favorable outcome, this does not appear to be the case. In one series of 33 patients who talked and then deteriorated to a GCS of 8 or less, the overall mortality rate was 45%; 76% of patients had intracranial hematomas, most of which were extra-axial, that were rapidly evacuated. Despite the aggressive approach, the mortality rate was 44%. A minority of patients in this series had signs of brain stem compression.

In our report of 100 patients with transtentorial herniation, 10 (77%) of 13 patients who had a transient lucid interval died despite burr-hole exploration and evacuation of intracranial mass lesions.[7] These results suggest that although a high initial GCS improves the likelihood of recovery, subsequent deterioration is a poor prognostic sign.

Residual Brain Stem Function

Abnormalities of pupillary function, extraocular movements, and patterns of motor response that indicate upper brain stem injury all predict a poor outcome after severe head injury.[6,8,11,12,18,21,26,27,33,41,42] In our series of 153 patients with transtentorial herniation, a good outcome or a moderate disability was significantly more common among patients with anisocoria than among those with bilaterally dilated and unreactive pupils (27% vs. 3.5%, $p < 0.05$) (see Chapter 7). Other reports have also shown that bilateral absence of pupillary function worsens the prognosis. In the series of Stone et al.,[42] 10 (25%) of 40 patients with a single dilated pupil ipsilateral to a subdural hematoma had a functional recovery, compared with only five (11%) of 44 patients with bilaterally absent pupillary function. Seelig et al.[41] reported that only six (10%) of 61 patients with severe upper brain stem dysfunction and bilaterally impaired pupillary and oculocephalic reflexes after severe head injury had a good outcome or a moderate disability. The loss of oculocephalic or oculovestibular reflexes combined with abnormal pupillary function indicates an even more profound depression of upper brain stem function and predicts a poor potential for recovery.[12,18,21,27] Marshall et al.[27] noted that only 14% of severely head-injured patients with impaired or absent oculocephalic reflexes had a good recovery, and 60% died.

Bricolo et al.[12] reviewed 800 patients with severe head injuries and reported that only 84% of those with bilateral extensor rigidity during their early hospital course died, and only 16% achieved a functional outcome. In contrast, the mortality rates were 57% among patients with bilateral flexor rigidity and 54% among those with unilateral abnormal motor responses.

The clinical signs of transtentorial herniation may improve after initial treatment with mannitol and hyperventilation or after evacuation of an intracranial mass lesion. Such improvement suggests that the clinical findings were more likely caused by the compressive effect of a mass lesion than by a primary injury to the brain stem. In such cases, the potential for functional recovery may be much greater than if the clinical signs persist after therapy. A unilateral third nerve palsy resulting from mechanical uncal herniation may require up to six weeks to improve after surgical decompression. Therefore, persistent anisocoria may have little prognostic importance in a patient who is otherwise showing clinical signs of recovering from a depressed level of consciousness and hemiparesis.

Multiple Injuries and Systemic Hypotension

The presence of additional injuries markedly worsens the potential for survival among head-injured patients.[30,32,33] Overgaard et al.[33] reported that thoracic or abdominal injury or extremity fractures significantly increased the mortality rate after moderate or severe head injury. A systolic blood pressure of 160 mm Hg or greater at admission correlated with increased morbidity and mortality rates in patients of all ages.

Systemic hypotension at admission is an extremely grave prognostic indicator. Miller et al.[30] reported that arterial hypotension, hypoxia, hypercarbia, and anemia were seen almost exclusively in patients with multiple systemic injuries in addition to severe head injury; this combination increased morbidity and mortality rates. In the series of Newfield et al.,[32] the mortality rate was 83% in severely head-injured patients who had systemic hypotension during the first 24 hours of hospitalization and 45% in those who did not ($p < 0.001$). Only three of 36 patients in our series who had hypotension and signs of transtentorial herniation at admission survived; no patient survived who had a systolic blood pressure less than 60 mm Hg or cardiac arrest at admission.[6]

Computerized Tomography

The findings on the initial CT scan can also help to predict the prognosis after severe head injury.[1,22,23,46,47,49] Lobato et al.[23] reported that patients whose CT scans were completely normal had a lower mortality rate and better functional recovery than patients whose scans showed abnormalities, even among patients with an initial GCS of 3 or 4, 26% of whom had a good outcome and 46% a moderate disability. In a later series,[22] these authors described 55 patients with diffuse hemispheric swelling; 94% of these patients had an ipsilateral extra-axial mass lesion, 82% had an initial GCS of 5 or less, and 74% had clinical signs of upper brain stem dysfunction. The mortality rate was 87%.

Compressed or obliterated basal cisterns on the initial CT scan may also worsen the clinical outcome. Toutant et al.[46] reported mortality rates of 22% in patients with normal-appearing basal cisterns, 39% in those with compressed cisterns, 77% in those with obliterated cisterns, and 100% in those with obliterated cisterns and a maximal midline shift greater than 15 mm. Obliterated cisterns were also associated with severe elevations of ICP. The predictive power of these CT findings was greater among patients with an initial GCS of 6 to 8 than among those with a GCS of 3 to 5. This suggests that increased ICP, mechanical brain displacement, and potential brain stem compression may be a more important cause of mortality in patients with a higher GCS than in those with a very low GCS, which reflects a more severe primary brain injury.

A hematoma on the initial CT scan may have prognostic importance. Severely head-injured patients with a subdural hematoma have a worse prognosis than those without an extra-axial mass lesion detected by CT.[15,22,23,46,47,49] We have found that clinical signs of transtentorial herniation at admission or within 12 hours were significantly more common in patients with temporal hematomas of 30 cc or larger than in patients with frontal or occipital hematomas of equal size.[5] Patients with temporal lobe hematomas had a significantly worse outcome than the other groups, and no patient with signs of transtentorial herniation had a good outcome (see Chapter 8). Hematomas of the brain stem (Duret hemorrhages) on CT scans after head injury[1,14] most often indicates severely increased intracranial pressure and transient downward herniation and ischemic injury of the brain stem (see Chapter 1). Such findings are generally associated with a poor prognosis for recovery.[14]

The type of lesion identified by CT also appears to influence the outcome and the extent of neuropsychological recovery after severe head injury. Uzzell et al.[47] reported that conscious survivors with diffuse swelling on early CT scans had higher levels of memory and learning ability than those with focal abnormalities; both groups had lower mortality rates than patients with evidence of diffuse axonal injury. Magnetic resonance (MR) imaging may identify lesions of the white matter and brain stem that are often missed on CT. The demonstration of widespread lesions by MR imaging predicts a poor prognosis for neurological recovery despite normal-appearing CT scans.[49]

Intracranial Pressure Monitoring

An abnormal increase in ICP and the ability to lower ICP with treatment correlate well with the overall prognosis for recovery and survival.[9,20,29,34,48] In 160 patients with severe head injury, few of whom had clinical signs of transtentorial herniation, Miller et al.[29] showed that any elevation of ICP was associated with increased morbidity. Patients who had and maintained a normal ICP had a mortality rate of 14%, and 78% eventually had a good outcome or moderate disability. Nearly half of those who died had severely elevated ICP at the time of initial measurement, and all patients with uncontrollably elevated ICP died. Pitts et al.[34] showed a significant linear relationship between the ICP 6 to 24 hours after injury and the outcome three months later. Among patients with an initial GCS of 3 to 5, Bowers and Marshall[10] showed that the survival rate was significantly greater if the ICP was monitored and elevations in ICP were treated.

Elevated ICP causes cerebral perfusion pressure (CPP) to decrease and thus results in cerebral ischemia. McGraw et al.[28] found that the sum of the average CPP and the lowest CPP predicted survival as effectively as ICP recording in approximately 98% of cases. Survival was less likely if the sum was less than 92 mm Hg.

Declaration of Brain Death

After transtentorial herniation, it is not uncommon that persistent and intractable elevation of ICP cause progression of severe injury to the brain, including the brain stem, despite maximal therapy. In this setting, there may be no clinical evidence of function in the cortical hemispheres or in the brain stem. Patients in this condition may fulfill the clinical requirements for the declaration of brain death.[34,36,43] Most states have passed a Uniform Determination of Death Act, under which patients who are declared brain dead have fulfilled the legal requirement for death regardless of whether they remain on life-support systems.[34]

The clinical criteria for declaration of death are (1) a known cause of CNS injury severe enough to account for the loss of brain function; (2) the absence of clinical factors that could depress the neurological examination, such as hypothermia, metabolic abnormalities, or CNS suppressant medications; and (3) the absence of all evidence of cortical and brain stem function. In most states, additional supportive tests are not necessary if all three criteria have been fulfilled. Useful ancillary tests that may confirm the presence and irreversibility of brain death include ICP monitoring[34,36,43] and measurements of cerebral blood flow using such techniques as angiography, radionuclide scans,[16] and transcranial Doppler ultrasound examination.[31] Irreversible brain death is confirmed if any of these tests demonstrates the lack of brain perfusion. Additional tests, such as electroencephalography[17] and somatosensory evoked potentials are less useful because they may be suppressed by metabolic and pharmacologic factors that suppress brain function.

It has been recommended that the irreversibility of apparent brain death can be confirmed by continued supportive care and observation.[34,36,43] The persistence of clinical evidence of brain death beyond 24 hours in an adult,[34,36] 48 hours in a child, and 72 hours in a neonate[43] is considered to confirm the irreversibility of brain death.

The declaration of brain death in appropriate clinical circumstances is important for several reasons. It serves to limit the unrealistic hopes of family and loved ones for the recovery of the patient. It also limits the continued use of expensive intensive care medical resources and potentially provides for organ donations. Often, the possibility of organ donation provides the only possible good that may result from an unfortunate tragedy. We strongly encourage the timely declaration of brain death in appropriate cases.

Summary

Although only a minority of patients with clinical signs of transtentorial herniation after head injury will survive, it is possible to predict with reasonable certainty the possibility for survival and a functional outcome. The prognosis is determined from the initial clinical examination, the radiological and surgical findings, and the early clinical course, and the results of ICP monitoring. The potential for a functional recovery is greater in younger patients; children in particular have a much greater likelihood not only for survival but also for a neurologically functional outcome. A higher initial GCS is another favorable sign; often, patients with the greatest chance for recovery have an initially high GCS that drops with the onset of clinical signs of transtentorial herniation. Patients likely to have a functional recovery almost always have some preservation of upper brain stem reflexes. Patients with bilaterally dilated and unreactive pupils, multiple injuries, initial systemic hypotension, or uncontrollably elevated ICP have a very poor prognosis.

Nevertheless, it remains difficult to predict with absolute certainty the potential for survival of individual patients, unless they have no cortical or brain stem function. When appropriate exclusionary criteria are observed,[34] these features reliably indicate brain death. In such cases, it is appropriate to plan to withdraw life support, and discuss with the family the concept of organ donation.[34] Among patients with some brain stem function, prognostic information is useful for realistic discussions with the family concerning the possibilities for survival and recovery. Management decisions can then be based on the clinical course of the patient and the perceptions of both the family and the treating physician.

References

1. Alexander E, Kushner J, Six EG: Brain stem hemorrhages and increased intracranial pressure: from Duret to computed tomography. Surg Neurol 17:107-110, 1982.
2. Alexandre A, Colombo F, Nertempi P, et al.: Cognitive outcome and early indices of severity of head injury. J Neurosurg 59: 751-761, 1983.
3. Amacher AL, Bybee DE: Toleration of head injury by the elderly. Neurosurgery 20:954-958, 1987.
4. Andrews BT: Management of delayed posttraumatic intracerebral hemorrhage. Contemp Neurosurg 10:1-6, 1988.
5. Andrews BT, Chiles BW, Olsen WL, et al.: The effect of intracerebral hematoma location on the risk of brain-stem compression and on clinical outcome. J Neurosurg 69:518-522, 1988.
6. Andrews BT, Levy ML, Pitts LH: The implications of systemic hypotension for the neurological examination in patients with severe head injury. Surg Neurol 28:419-422, 1987.
7. Andrews BT, Pitts LH, Lovely MP, et al.: Is computed tomographic scanning necessary in patients with tentorial herniation? Results of immediate surgical exploration without computed tomography in 100 patients. Neurosurgery 19:408-414, 1986.
8. Becker DP, Miller JD, Ward JD, et al.: The outcome from severe head injury with early diagnosis and intensive management. J Neurosurg 47:491-502, 1977.
9. Berger MS, Pitts LH, Lovely M, et al.: Outcome from severe head injury in children and adolescents. J Neurosurg 62:194-199, 1985.
10. Bowers SA, Marshall LF: Outcome in 200 consecutive cases of severe head injury treated in San Diego County: a prospective analysis. Neurosurgery 6:237-241, 1980.
11. Brender SJ, Selverstone B: Recovery from decerebration. Brain 93:381-392, 1970.
12. Bricolo A, Turazzi S, Alexandre A, et al.: Decerebrate rigidity in acute head injury. J Neurosurg 47:680-698, 1977.

13. Bruce DA, Schut L, Bruno L, et al.: Outcome following severe head injuries in children. J Neurosurg 48:679-688, 1978.
14. Cooper PR, Maravilla K, Kirkpatrick J, et al.: Traumatically induced brain stem hemorrhages and the computerized tomographic scan: clinical, pathological, and experimental observations. Neurosurgery 4:115-124, 1979.
15. Gennarelli TA, Spielman GM, Langfitt TW, et al.: Influence of the type of intracranial lesion on outcome from severe head injury—a multicenter study using a new classification system. J Neurosurg 56:26-32, 1982.
16. Goodman JM, Heck LL, Moore BD: Confirmation of brain death with portable isotope angiography. A review of 204 consecutive cases. Neurosurgery 16:492-497, 1985.
17. Grigg MM, Kelly MA, Celesia GG, et al.: Electroencephalographic activity after brain death. Arch Neurol 44:948-954, 1987.
18. Gutterman P, Shenken HA: Prognostic features in recovery from decerebration. J Neurosurg 32:330-335, 1979.
19. Hoff JT, Spetzler R, Winestock D: Head injury and early signs of tentorial herniation—a management dilemma. West J Med 128: 112-116, 1978.
20. Jamieson KG, Yelland JD: Surgically treated traumatic subdural hematomas. J Neurosurg 37:137-149, 1972.
21. Jennett B, Teasdale G, Braakman R, et al.: Prognosis of patients with severe head injury. Neurosurgery 4:283-289, 1979.
22. Lobato RD, Sarabia R, Cordobes F, et al.: Posttraumatic cerebral hemispheric swelling: analysis of 55 cases studied with computerized tomography. J Neurosurg 68:417-423, 1988.
23. Lobato RD, Sarabia R, Rivas JJ, et al.: Normal computerized tomography scans in severe head injury. Prognostic and clinical implications. J Neurosurg 65:784-789, 1986.
24. Lokkeberg AR, Grimes RM: Assessing the influence of non-treatment variables in a study of outcome from severe head injuries. J Neurosurg 61:254-262, 1984.
25. Luerssen TG, Klauber MR, Marshall LF: Outcome from head injury related to patient's age. A longitudinal prospective study of adults and pediatric head injury. J Neurosurg 68:409-416, 1988.
26. Marshall LF, Barba D, Toole BM, et al.: Oval pupil: clinical significance and relationship to intracranial hypertension. J Neurosurg 58:566-568, 1983.

27. Marshall LF, Smith RW, Shapiro HM: The outcome with aggressive treatment in severe head injuries. Part 1: the significance of intracranial pressure monitoring. J Neurosurg 50:20-25, 1979.
28. McGraw C, Shields CB, Gamel JW, et al.: Impact of cerebral perfusion pressure on survival following head injury. In Miller JD, Teasdale GM, Rowan LO, et al. (eds): Intracranial Pressure VI. Berlin: Springer-Verlag, 1986, pp 667-670.
29. Miller JD, Becker DP, Ward JD, et al.: Significance of intracranial hypertension in severe head injury. J Neurosurg 47:503-516, 1977.
30. Miller JD, Sweet RC, Narayan R, et al.: Early insults to the injured brain. JAMA 240:439-442, 1978.
31. Newell DW, Grady MS, Sirotta P, et al.: Evaluation of brain death using transcranial Doppler. Neurology 24:509-513, 1989.
32. Newfield P, Pitts L, Kaktis J, et al.: Influence of shock on survival after head injury. Neurosurgery 6:596-597, 1980.
33. Overgaard J, Christensen S, Hvid-Hansen O, et al.: Prognosis after head injury based on early clinical examination. Lancet 2:7830-7835, 1973.
34. Pitts LH: Determination of brain death. West J Med 140:628-631, 1984.
35. Pitts LH, Kaktis JV, Juster R, et al.: ICP and outcome in patients with severe head injury. In Shulman K, Marmarou A, Miller JD, et al. (eds): Intracranial Pressure IV. Berlin: Springer-Verlag, 1980, pp 5-9.
36. President's Commission Report: Guidelines for the Determination of Death. JAMA 246:2184-2188, 1981.
37. Richards T, Hoff J: Factors affecting survival from acute subdural hematoma. Surgery 75:253-258, 1974.
38. Rockswold GL: Reply to letter: Management of closed head injury patients who "talked and deteriorated." Neurosurgery 22: 614, 1988.
39. Rockswold GL, Leonard PR, Nagib MG: Analysis of management in thirty-three closed head injury patients who "talked and deteriorated." Neurosurgery 21:51-55, 1987.
40. Seelig JM, Becker DP, Miller JD, et al.: Traumatic acute subdural hematoma-major mortality reduction in comatose patients treated within four hours. N Engl J Med 304:1511-1517, 1981.
41. Seelig JM, Greenberg RP, Becker DP, et al.: Reversible brain stem dysfunction following acute traumatic subdural hematoma—a

clinical and electrophysiological study. J Neurosurg 55:516-523, 1981.

42. Stone JL, Rifai MHS, Surgar O, et al.: Subdural hematomas I: acute subdural hematoma: progress in definition, clinical pathology and therapy. Surg Neurol 19:216-231, 1983.
43. Task Force for Determination of Brain Death in Children: Guidelines for the determination of brain death in children. Arch Neurol 44:587-590, 1987.
44. Teasdale G, Jennett B: Assessment of coma and impaired consciousness: a practical scale. Lancet 2:81-84, 1974.
45. Teasdale G, Skene A, Parker L, et al.: Age and outcome of severe head injury. Acta Neurochir (Suppl) 28:140-143, 1979.
46. Toutant SM, Klauber MR, Marshall LF, et al.: Absent or compressed basal cisterns on first CT scan: ominous predictors of outcome in severe head injury. J Neurosurg 61:691-694, 1984.
47. Uzzell BP, Dolinkas CA, Wiser RF, et al.: Influence of lesions detected by computed tomography on outcome and neuropsychological recovery after severe head injury. Neurosurgery 20: 396-402, 1987.
48. Uzzell BP, Obrist WD, Dolinkas CA, et al.: Relationship of acute CBF and ICP findings to neuropsychological outcome in severe head injury. J Neurosurg 65:630-635, 1986.
49. Wilberger JE, Deeb Z, Rothfus W: Magnetic resonance imaging in cases of severe head injury. Neurosurgery 20:571-576, 1987.
50. Williams JM, Gomes F, Drudge OW, et al.: Predicting outcome from closed head injury by early assessment of trauma. J Neurosurg 61:581-585, 1984.

Index